The Anthropology of Alternative Medicine

The Anthropology of Alternative Medicine

Anamaria Iosif Ross

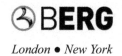

London • New York

English edition
First published in 2012 by
Berg
Editorial offices:
50 Bedford Square, London, W1CB 3DP, UK
175 Fifth Avenue, New York, NY 10010, USA

Berg is an imprint of Bloomsbury Publishing Plc.

Library of Congress Cataloging-in-Publication Data

A catalogue record for this book is available from the Library of Congress.

British Library Cataloguing-in-Publication Data

A catalogue record for this book is available from the British Library.

ISBN 978 1 84520 801 1 (Cloth)
978 1 84520 802 8 (Paper)

Typeset by Apex CoVantage, LLC, Madison, WI, USA
Printed in the UK by the MPG Books Group

www.bergpublishers.com

*To my mother Valentina and my sons
Benjamin Luca and Maxwell Toma,
for the motivation and encouragement
to delight, explore, and persist in my dreams*

Contents

Acknowledgments

This book would not have happened without the inspiration and support of many extraordinary people who have graciously provided me with their wisdom, assistance, and understanding over the years. My research interest in "alternative medicine" was encouraged at Tulane University by the distinguished scholars Victoria Bricker, Adeline Masquelier, and William Balée. It was brought to life by generous informants, friends, and colleagues through their willingness to include my interests and queries into their lives.

I especially wish to thank writer Vasile Andru, ELTA founder Ion Dumitrescu, Dr. Lucian Stratan, and the ELTA members who shared their insights and resources with me. The time spent with practitioners, supporters, and advocates of alternative medicine or *medicină naturistă* in Romania has been provocative and nourishing in countless ways. My Romanian fieldwork was generously supported by a junior Fulbright grant, and the writing of the original dissertation by a Selley Fellowship at Tulane. In Romania, I was generously welcomed and greatly assisted by the energetic and insightful scholars at the *Francisc I. Rainer Anthropological Research Institute* in Bucharest: Ioan Oprescu, Cornelia Guja, Radu Răutu, and Cristiana Glavce, the Institute's tireless director.

The coming-into-the-world of this book must be credited to the elegant and perceptive Anna Wright, my Berg editor, who navigated my ups and downs during the past three years with the poise of a seasoned Tai Chi master. Her gentle but firm encouragement and feedback have been immeasurably helpful and reassuring in the journey from proposal to print. The idea for this book belongs to the spirited Hanna Shakespeare, my first editor at Berg, who first envisioned my writing such a book on the basis of our conversations about my Romanian fieldwork, and who guided me expertly through the proposal process. Mary Drucker and her husband David Drucker provided invaluable wisdom and editing suggestions in the final stages. Karina Ross generously lent her attentive eye to the proofs.

The writing of this book has been a logistical adventure, since shortly after starting the project my family expanded with the joyful arrival of our second child. My immense gratitude goes to my husband David Ross and my vivacious boys, Ben and Max, for their love, help, sacrifice, and tolerance as I have struggled to carve out the time needed for this project at a time when David was actively pursuing his own Ph.D. and scholarly work on creativity. I am deeply thankful to my generous family in Romania: Luminiţa Blănaru, Coca Andronescu, Ovidiu Gartig, Tamara

Gartig, Steluţa si Alecu Miu, as well as my dear friends and colleagues Cristina Păiş Montgomery, Alicia DeVora, Lisa Orr, Jo Ellen Vespo, Melodee Moltman, Sherri Cash, Su-Lien Miller, Angel and Naybell Rivera, John and Margarita Foreman, Ajsa Korajac, Alice and Cătălin Butunoi, Kim and Orin Domenico, Stacey Giroux Wells, Jonathan Barns, Atasi Basu, Tejashree Sayanak, Simone Shaheen, Diane Nickerson de Feliz, and Danhong Zhang, who gave me strength during challenging times in my life and career. My father, Dr. George Yossif, has modeled life-long curiosity, passion, and courage in learning and thinking, which I hope will equally inspire my talented young brother Oliver Yossif on his journeys.

The hope and resilience that permeate this book are a tribute to my gentle and luminous mother Valentina Iosif, née Valentina Blănaru, and to my grandmothers Steluţa Blănaru and Eugenia Yossif, whose complete devotion to their families and inexhaustible passion for life remain my invisible anchors.

Alternative Medicine in the Twenty-First Century

Alternative medicine is ideally suited to anthropological examination, being commonly represented as the elusive and challenging *other* of modern capitalist biomedical systems. It is an eclectic array of healing resources, methods, and practitioners that exist mostly outside the dominant system of health care of a particular society at a particular point in time. Since the label *alternative medicine* means a multitude of things in different contexts, it is a unique challenge to define and explore its diverse approaches and social interconnections, particularly in a brief yet multifaceted manner that addresses a broad audience that includes health professionals, university students, and novice scholars of holistic healing. This book takes on the timely task of providing a concentrated anthropological synthesis at a time when diverse "complementary and alternative therapies" (known in biomedical circles under the acronym CAM) have been steadily gaining visibility and acceptance, becoming gradually integrated into the mainstream of health systems in many parts of the contemporary world, and playing a progressively significant role in the social relations of health care (Cant and Sharma 1999; Baer 2001; Keegan 2001; Ernst 2002; Whorton 2002; Lee-Treweek et al. 2005).

For millennia, diverse approaches to healing have coexisted and blended through time and space, often as a result of cultural contact. The extreme dominance of Western medicine during the twentieth century is an atypical historical event. The view that *biomedicine* (twentieth-century Western allopathic medicine based in biological science) should be the only legitimate healing practice was a vision of modern rationalism that has not become realized. While it has been growing in popularity in recent decades, alternative healing is not a newly fashionable trend but a well-established cultural strategy and a dynamic, heterogeneous feature of most contemporary medical landscapes: a way in which people seek to maximize their chances for well-being and adapt to rapidly changing or unfavorable circumstances, drawing on multiple sources and resources of knowledge and authority. At the same time, there are some powerful new trends at work, such as the increased consumption and commercialization of unconventional healing methods, a growing trend toward the professionalization of alternative and complementary practitioners, the integration of biomedicine with alternative medicine, and the growing impact of globalization and the Internet. The latter is involved in creating, reviving, or promoting alternative healing communities, lifestyles, methods, and products for healing that are inter-connected with the increasing commoditization of foods, medicines, wellness, and spirituality.

The anthropological quest for interpretations of alien cultural experiences is itself a "therapeutic quest for meaning, a search for identity that can be considered a form of healing in the broadest sense," wrote Loring Danforth (1989:300). The modern health-seeker's path through the realm of healing alternatives resembles the anthro-pologist's journey through distant landscapes and customs, a journey driven by the hope of achieving a new coherence, a more meaningful narrative of suffering and the human condition, and an enabling transformation of our vulnerable (and often marginal) identity in a much larger context. Like a modern fieldwork site, the world of alternative healing practices is highly dynamic and elusive, subject to multiple cri-tiques and interpretations, at once inviting and forbidding to the incidental observer. It may not be pinned down or taxonomized in a classic ethnographic or sociological manner. The emergent contours of alternative medicine can only be fleetingly cap-tured in the shifting mirrors of modern life experience, health politics, and globaliza-tion. There are discernible themes and patterns at work, but practices and participants are not fixed, and boundaries are easily blurred.

Multitudes of unrelated and profoundly different approaches to healing are com-monly lumped together by consumers, the mass media, governments, and health professionals under this generous umbrella term, including herbal treatments that are millennia old, the latest raw-food diets that challenge the hygienic imperatives of capitalist public health policies, and religious rituals that posit an essential role for the soul within the complex processes of health, illness, and healing. While it is considered a valid designation in the popular imagination, it is impossible to distin-guish with certainty what alternative medicine is and what it is not, or where it be-gins and where it ends, especially now that, with the advent of the third millennium and the communicative power of the Internet, the overlap and integration of various alternatives with biomedicine seems to be increasing throughout the industrialized world. Nina Etkin (2006:204) aptly observed: "Depending on one's perspective, CAM is a category of exclusion, preventive and therapeutic modalities that fall out-side the conventional U.S. medical practice, or a category of inclusion, a residuum of everything else, ranging widely from prayer to acupuncture to Ayurvedic plant medicines."

Without a doubt, alternative medicine is a dynamic and evolving field, and if one may call it a field at all, it is only in the sense of a *conceptual* field that re-quires the continual labors of popular imagination and authoritative discourses for its existence. The medicine of the nineteenth century was highly pluralistic throughout the world. Baer (2001) described practitioners of "regular" (ortho-dox) and "irregular" (heterodox) medicine in the United States as competing in a weakly regulated social landscape in which the proponents of contrasting systems of healing described one another in mutually hostile terms. Orthodox medicine descended from the "heroic medicine" of the colonial era, which endorsed aggressive measures such as sweating, purging, and toxic drugs. It contrasted with the practices and views of heterodox medicine "sects" of the time, which tended to uphold gentler methods and the view that healing involved strengthening one's vital force and required more than just mechanistic interventions (Baer 2001:7–8). These nineteenth-century healing systems included homeopathy, botanic medicine, hydropathy, osteopathy, chiropractic, Christian Science, and folk healing, some of which were further divided into various subgroupings with specific professional training and associations.

Impressive achievements in infectious disease control, particularly the advent of germ theory, the discovery of antibiotics, and the creation of vaccines, inaugurated a century-long era of hegemonic authority and cultural prominence of biophysical reductionism in Western capitalist societies. In the early part of this century, scientific medicine represented in the United States by the American Medical Association (AMA) successfully asserted extensive dominance both politically and economically on all other health practitioners, establishing itself as the lead arbiter of medical orthodoxy, effectiveness, and validity in American health care. Similarly, biomedical practitioners in other capitalist societies, such as Great Britain and Australia, achieved dominance over heterodox practitioners and acted to restrict their rights and monopolize funding (Singer and Baer 2007:129). Nevertheless, unorthodox alternatives survived, and some even thrived through these times of marginalization, often wielding significant political power and defying political and cultural categories. Although they were contested in the United States via complex webs of interest-group rivalries and political power struggles, Robert D. Johnston (2004:2) notes that the regime of alternatives was not entirely "frozen in social and intellectual disrepute." Although much changed in the twentieth century, on a deeper level, much remained the same: the diversity of practices was not extinguished and neither was the desire for democracy in the health care arena, in the form of multiple choices and the rights of minorities to live according to their values and pursue their aims. The practice and use of nonbiomedical therapies has always deeply been tied to class and ethnic distinctions and relations, and is therefore a highly political process. As twentieth-century scientific medicine became increasingly characterized by commercialism and corporatization, traditional and unconventional health movements and practices became prominent venues of cultural criticism, resistance, and empowerment in many parts of the world (Johnston 2004; Ross 2003; Klassen 2001).

Ideas and practices, old and new, flow in and out of the alternative medicine sphere as they gain or lose credibility, power, and prestige in the pragmatic and interconnected worlds of biomedical and clinical research, health policy, and economic solvency. An example of this nexus constitutes the transformation of the Chinese star anise plant, traditionally used in Asian medicine and cooking (being a key ingredient in five-spice powder), into the expensive and elaborately produced pharmaceutical drug Tamiflu, which shortens the course of flu and other viral illnesses. The high-technology processing and global commodification of a traditional ingredient by a multinational pharmaceutical company created temporary shortages of star anise, as governments began stockpiling the drug, until manufacturers discovered an alternate way to produce the active ingredient (shikimic acid) using the fermentation of bacterium *E. coli*. The cost of the spice (commonly used in Chinese stews) rose significantly after the 2009 swine flu outbreak (Lim 2009).

What constitutes the mainstream at one particular time, like the use of leeches by physicians in the eighteenth and nineteenth centuries, may be considered questionable and/or alternative a century later. The use of leeches was discredited by modern sensibilities and usurped by newer methods and technologies but ascended to the status of cutting-edge medical science again at the dawn of the twenty-first century. Recently, plastic surgeons have begun to use leeches to relieve the blood engorgement and swelling of skin grafts; hygienic medical maggots are being used to clean dead tissue from wounds and prevent the onset of gangrene; pig whipworm eggs are voluntarily ingested to modulate overactive immune systems and induce remission for Crohn's bowel disease: these parasites are now part of modern biomedical science. These zoo-therapies, reminiscent of the Dark Ages, seem to work better than any modern technologies at hand. An analogous phenomenon is the resurgence of saltwater rinses and gargles for inflamed sinuses or throats, a traditional home remedy that Indo-European grandmothers had been using for millennia, which is now recommended by physicians alongside modern drugs and surgeries. There lies refreshing irony in the fact that such old-fashioned methods of healing are being reclaimed by modern medical science and health care at a time when the pace of scientific advancement and discovery in medicine is faster and more awe-inspiring than ever.

Not only does the passage of time play odd tricks on the notion of "alternative"—so does space. Geographically, practices that originate elsewhere are more commonly viewed as alternative, at least until they gain common currency. This is sometimes due to lesser availability of practitioners, increased cost of therapies, or limited social authority and recognition. The use of probiotic supplements and homeopathic medicines by mainstream health providers is becoming increasingly common and accepted in Europe but still remains questioned or marginalized within the U.S. medical world as something yet insufficiently proven. More than three thousand years old, Traditional Chinese Medicine (TCM) is fully accepted in China, where it is widely used alongside modern Western medicine, yet it is still considered alternative in Europe and the United States, although its health benefits are increasingly supported by scientific data.

The gold standard of evidence-based research in the Western medical world remains represented by double-blind placebo-controlled medical trials, involving thousands of participants, which are elaborate and expensive to organize, monitor, and interpret accurately. This challenge is particularly difficult for alternative therapies,

What about Studies/Trials

even time-tested ancient ones, supported by millennia of cultural experience, primarily because of high costs of the biomedical research methods in terms of time and money. At the governmental level, resources devoted to "alternative medicine research" have until recently been nonexistent and continue to be paltry in comparison to those devoted to mainstream biomedical research. Scientists working with ideas and models that challenge the dominant theories have traditionally been discriminated against in terms of financial support and ostracized in scientific communities in the Western world. However, the tide has started to turn, and modern scientific testing methods have recently begun to be applied to a number of traditional and alternative therapies with encouraging results, from laboratory studies of traditional herbal remedies to MRI and neurophysiology studies of healing practices like meditation, music therapy and qigong. Not surprisingly, Western scientific medicine is currently quite the alternative *other* in most remote and impoverished areas of the world, where it is regarded as a last resort, due to lack of accessibility and great cost relative to local resources. In less developed communities, home remedies and traditional medicines (particularly those made from locally grown plants) continue to provide the majority of healing and constitute the first line of therapy (Bussmann and Sharon 2006). *how many other likes?*

Indeed, what is deemed alternative at a particular time and place is often a mainstream practice in another time and place. Users and providers of remedies, along with governmental and administrative authorities do not tend to share the same meanings. It is significant that *alter* means "other" in Latin, as in the expression *alter ego* (which can mean a second self, a trusted friend, or the opposite side of a personality) and that the notion of alternative references the idea of choice, most commonly between mutually exclusive possibilities, as well as "different from the usual or conventional: existing or functioning outside the established cultural, social, or economic system" (Merriam-Webster's Online Dictionary 2010). This captures the elusive social spirit of alternative medicine: its subversive and grassroots qualities, the lack of formulaic standardization, and the fact that authorities have devoted significant energy and resources to making sure that alternatives maintain lesser status, power and social recognition either alongside or within the margins of dominant systems.

The verb "to alternate" points to a back and forth motion, recalling the undulating sine wave used to represent alternative electrical current, a fluid movement between two opposite poles or values that passes through every possible value in between. In a social context where multiple healing modalities are present or possible, the search for health care can be visualized as a "probability wave," described in quantum physics. Selecting a particular healing method or set of methods "collapses the wave," instantiating one concrete experiential reality or blending of options. The wavelike nature of this movement refers to the fact that the ill person and his or her family may choose only a formal biomedical approach, an informal home-based approach, or any combination of biomedical and nonbiomedical healing practices.

The multiple permutations of therapeutic options that exist in most contemporary settings are limited in every local context by particular (social and personal) boundaries and constraints, such as the resources of time, money, transportation or information. In addition, it is meaningful to note that the action verb "to alter" means to change, modify or transform. Like "to alternate," it captures the dynamism that characterizes healing in real-world settings. As healers and patients seek to change a condition of illness and transform it into well-being, improvement, comfort or acceptance, they appropriate and deploy the language, symbols and methods of particular medical traditions and distinctive social settings, making their efforts and quests authoritative and relevant in a social field of action and interaction. When someone (patient or healer) declares that a hernia has been repaired, an energy blockage has been removed, or a bad spirit has been appeased or driven away, specific cultural models and cultural realities are invoked, restoring a sense of order and bringing emotional and logical relief, based on mutual trust and understandings.

The heterogeneity of "alternative medicine" makes it difficult and potentially misleading to study as one distinct entity, as the many eclectic practices and traditions that come under this designation have emerged from and represent diverse cultural histories and worldviews. In light of this, Cant and Sharma (1999:5) suggest that the plural term alternative *medicines* is more appropriate than the singular. While I agree with their observation, upon acknowledging the heterogeneous and multiple nature of the object, it is reasonable to employ the singular, with the understanding that it functions as a collective noun, reflecting a fragmented, diverse, and pluralistic reality. I consider the title of "alternative medicine" or the more favored contemporary designation of CAM to be a useful yet highly problematic category for the purposes of this book. Therefore, the notion of *alternative* will be used cautiously and its contextual meanings will be interrogated often.

At all times, the reader is called on to recognize the contingent, provisional, and emergent nature of this cultural label, which entails complex cultural baggage even when none is apparent. What is considered "alternative" depends not only on one's perspective and social position but also on historical, political, and economic circumstances that cause power and authority to infuse a particular set of practices or practitioners, which may become institutionalized as the mainstream. In many ethnographic settings this term is not really applicable, as real-world healing options and practices can defy simple categorizations and polarities, blending elements and practices of folk medicine with biomedicine and various other approaches. A contemporary work on healing must also acknowledge the major impact of political economy and globalization on patterns of health, illness, and health seeking. Sickness and suffering are not just natural processes: they are socially produced and shaped by local and global patterns of social inequality and power relations. Alternative healing is inextricably bound up into these relations as well, expressing, appropriating, embodying, redistributing, or challenging power and authority.

Conflicting Interests Pertaining to the Rise of Integrative Medicine

All therapeutic alternatives do not work equally well for all persons or for all ailments, nor do they have comparable records of safety, effectiveness, or popularity.
Whereas in India, China, and Japan traditional medicine has long been significant
and valued part of health care, in Western countries it is just beginning to gain recognition. Authoritative scholars and institutions in the United States, United Kingdom, Australia, and other nations have spearheaded rigorous scientific studies of
the benefits of various "unconventional" methods, evaluating and incorporating alternatives into mainstream medical practice. This revival of interest has led to the
creation of entities such as the National Center for Complementary and Alternative
Medicine (NCCAM) of the National Institutes of Health (NIH) in 1998 (established
initially as the Office of Alternative Medicine in 1991) in the United States and the
Research Council for Complementary Medicine (RCCM) in the United Kingdom,
university-based centers, such as Harvard's Center for Holistic Pediatric Education
and Research (CHPER), as well as professional associations, such as the Australian
Integrative Medicine Association, formed in 1992, later expanded into the Austral-
asian Integrative Medicine Association (Baer 2008).

David Eisenberg, the lead author of a highly influential article published in the
New England Journal of Medicine, found that one in three Americans use some form
of alternative medicine and make more visits to unconventional therapy providers
than to primary care physicians (Eisenberg et al. 1993). Yet most people do not discuss their use of unorthodox practices with their caregivers. The Eisenberg study
quickly rose to prominence in medical and CAM research communities, and the
article became widely quoted as support for the vitality and relevance of unconventional therapies in the United States. Cant and Sharma (1999) point to this study and
comparable English and Australian studies indicating that popular appeal of alternative medicines and practitioners is enormous and accounts for substantial and rapidly
increasing expenditures; they also note that, while there is less data from Southern
and Eastern Europe, existing evidence suggests that the pattern there is analogous.
Former communist countries experienced an efflorescence of nonbiomedical methods and practitioners since the fall of communism, but ethnographic studies have
shown that traditional practices and beliefs involving health, illness, and healing
were never fully extinguished (Lindquist 2006; Ross 2003).

As interest and concern regarding the increasing use of holistic and integrative
therapies has emerged to the fore in biomedical circles (most forcefully in the United
States and the United Kingdom), a number of authoritative debunkers and skeptics
have decried and denounced recent trends, claiming that the popularity and effectiveness claims made by Eisenberg et al. on behalf of CAM used flawed and deceptive
data, including things such as commercial weight-loss clinics and common home
remedies in their tabulations (Gorski 1999). Another vocal critic, William M. London
(2006), argued that there is no legitimate category of health care called "alternative

medicine," the reputation of which is much inflated by propaganda, profiteering, and the cheery personal anecdotes of enthusiasts: "it is a mere marketing label promoted as if it were a medical specialty." He prefers to refer to it as "so-called complementary and alternative medicine (sCAM)" and insists that there is little scientific evidence that alternative therapies provide more than symptomatic relief, despite their growing popularity and mainstreaming: they are simply unproven.

An academic clinical neurologist at Yale University School of Medicine, Steven Novella (2007), exemplifies an enlightened skeptical view of the CAM phenomenon. Novella is co-founder of the New England Skeptical Society, and producer of the weekly podcast titled "The Skeptics' Guide to the Universe" and the blog "Science-Based Medicine." He says that medical science and its institutions are under siege by antiscientific philosophy and the defenders of scientific medicine are treated as ideologues. Agreeing with Stephen Barrett, founder of Quackwatch.com, whom he recently interviewed, Novella believes that we are living in "a golden age of quackery," a time pseudoscience is becoming legitimized in medicine, exemplified by creation of NCCAM within the NIH. He compares the social infrastructures being created to support such pseudoscience to metastatic cancer: once it has spread may be difficult or impossible to eradicate. Similar critiques are expressed by biomedical skeptics in Australia, many of whom are members of an organization called Australian Skeptics, Incorporated (Baer 2008:60–1).

To the dismay of bioscientific purists, whose polemics discount alternative healing methods as relying on "anecdotal" evidence, and contrast it with the "evidence-based" approaches touted as the basis of biomedicine, integrative approaches to healing are rapidly gaining appeal with biomedical practitioners and consumers of health services and products on the global market. Medical schools and professional programs in the United States and United Kingdom are increasingly providing familiarization courses on alternative therapies and the impact of culturally diverse beliefs and practices on health, illness, and health care experiences; although movement in this direction has been slower in Australia, there too medical and nursing schools have begun to include a CAM component in their curriculum (Baer 2008; CU School of Medicine 2011). Mainstream health practitioners and institutions are increasingly eager to co-opt holistic and alternative practices, recognizing their tremendous economic potential and the positive impact they appear to have on patient loyalty and satisfaction (CUMC 2009a, 2009b; Dream Online 2009). However, governments are eager to assess and regulate these practices, which can provide additional sources of income (through licensing, for example) and novel cost-containment solutions, as the costs of high-tech and pharma-driven medicine continue to soar.

Hans Baer (2001) observed that several dangers result from this mainstreaming of CAM, chiefly the loss of the self-help and grass-roots ethos that have historically characterized alternative therapies, rendering their use into an increasingly upper-class phenomenon. As practices become professionalized, bureaucratized, and commercialized, they may become luxuries for the wealthy. After a century of net biomedical domination and systemic marginalization of unorthodox therapies, the rise of integrative medicine can be viewed as a strategy of domination *via* incorporation from the perspective of unconventional and traditional practitioners, who have been functioning outside the bureaucracy of health systems. Many traditionally trained healers are understandably ambivalent about the prospect of physicians, nurses, and other mainstream health practitioners acquiring training and licenses in hybrid but inauthentic fields such as "oriental medicine," so that they can compete in the market.

What Distinguishes an Anthropological Approach to Alternative Healing?

A question that needs to be addressed from the beginning is this: how is the approach featured herein different from that found in popular books, which present alternative medicine as a modern consumer product, cultural phenomenon, or timely trend to tap into? It is anthropological: thus, it embraces the culturally complicated and the inherent interdisciplinarity of the topic, together with the contingent nature of theories, practices, and experiences of healing. Without going into great technical or historical detail for each healing modality, this work explores diverse popular methods and ideas in cultural context, rather than abstractly, as isolated objects or summaries of facts. It seeks to explore and clarify the value and meaning that alternative medical approaches contribute to the lives of patients, practitioners, and communities, and how these alternative etiologies and therapeutic methods are constructed, imagined, or contested in time and space. This perspective seeks to communicate and validate the cultural experiences and testimonies of people and populations who employ or practice nonbiomedical therapies, rather than prove or disprove their objective validity in quantitative terms, although a certain amount of vetting or advocacy may inevitably co-occur, as well. Culturally speaking, practices and beliefs endure because they have social power, they fulfill needs and they yield benefits. These can be cognitive, emotional, social, material, or physical; patterns of benefit may not be statistically relevant in a numerical sense. As long as a healing approach endures and becomes perpetuated, it has significance, merit, value, and relevance from a social and anthropological perspective.

Dominant Themes and Organization of the Book

Several broad themes are explored throughout the book, as summarized further on. Each chapter tends to predominantly highlight one theme, but the themes are fundamentally intertwined. Western medical, communicative, and institutional practices commonly separate substance from energy from information, while they compartmentalize bodies, minds, spirit(s), and diverse sense perceptions into tidy and distinct categories of experience, therapeutics, and analysis. But the boundaries between these domains are permeable, if not illusory. Taking our categories for natural facts entails distortions and misrepresentations of how health, illness, and healing take place as phenomena. They are not separable, experientially or analytically, any more than the futures of persons, families, or communities could ever be fully separated from their pasts.

1. Diverse approaches to health, illness, and healing engage mindful, social, and political bodies across shifting, permeable, impermanent boundaries of persons, ideas, practices.
2. Flow and circulation are central to biological and social life, wellness, and healing: they are ecological phenomena, experiential realities, and metaphorical tools for thought.
3. Healing experiences are mediated through emotion, inter-relation, movement, and sensual experience, while being grounded in local contexts and interpretations.
4. The senses act and interact with the world in ways that are dynamic and complex: their role in healing goes much beyond current Western conceptions and approaches.

This introduction lays down the book's dominant concerns and assumptions, interrogates the meanings of the "alternative" label, and provides a brief overview of key anthropological concepts pertinent to the study of health and healing. The second chapter explores the significance of flow and circulation of substances, energy, and information as environmental, physiological, and analytical experiences directly implicated in health and healing across individual, local, and global dimensions. This chapter includes my own ethnographic reflections on the group ELTA Universitate, a millennial movement that I explored during my 1998 work in Romania, supported by a Fulbright grant. The third chapter addresses the role of consciousness in healing, drawing on a diversity of examples and accounts, including the practice of Hesychast prayer in Romania, to illustrate the variety of conceptions of mind/soul/spirit and the unique ways in which diverse therapies and healing traditions address the role of spirit(s) and consciousness in health and healing. The fourth and last chapter surveys the importance of sensory experiences (touch, smell, taste, movement, color) across various healing traditions, as well as my own experience with becoming initiated into Real Reiki in Romania. For young scholars, health professions students, and undergraduate students in anthropology, each chapter contains a list of further readings and films, reflection questions, and Internet sources, which may assist the faculty member or the student in journeying deeper into the world of alternative medicine, exploring personal biases and interpretations, or seeking diverse media for enhancing learning, critical thinking, and reflection.

Every subtopic or example addressed in the book arguably would deserve a chapter or a book of its own, which may at times disappoint a seasoned reader or frustrate the avid novice. But it is the risky nature of such a writing task, which seeks to be adventurous as well as concise and open-ended. As it succeeds in cutting an interdisciplinary streak through a wide range of contemporary scholarship and popular works on complementary and alternative medical practices, many of which are creative blendings of multiple traditions, it will at times seem haphazard or even unjust in its selections, and peculiar in its emphases, whetting the appetite for more local details, touching too briefly on many worthy topics, omitting some influential scholars. I wholeheartedly apologize in advance to the remarkable scholars, cultures, or therapies that have been weakly represented or marginalized. They would have surely enriched this account in a great number of ways.

Anthropology and the Human Journey

While it may be tempting to think of cultural diversity and interaction as recent hallmarks of globalization and multiculturalism in the third millennium, they are probably much older than histories and civilizations. Sociocultural variation (and possibly the awareness of it) goes back as far as the dawn of human cultures, 30,000 to 100,000 years ago, or some time before that, when communities of anatomically modern humans and Neanderthals shared the Earth, developing distinct material cultures and communication systems. Coexistence and interbreeding may have occurred, with Neanderthal genes surviving after extinction of Neanderthals around 30,000 B.C.E. Current genomic research shows that present-day Eurasians carry more Neanderthal genetic variants than sub-Saharan Africans alive today (Green et al. 2010). Indeed, the world has been a melting pot for much longer than it is commonly acknowledged. Detailed accounts of the life-ways and beliefs of diverse peoples were written down by the Greek scholar Herodotus in the fifth century B.C.E., and by the Persian scholar Al-Biruni, more than 1,000 years ago. The history of diversity continues in the ancient and medieval worlds of Europe and Asia, from the Barbarian invasions of Roman colonies to the many uneasy alliances forged within and without the Byzantine and Ottoman empires. Therein, many cultures and religions coexisted, often harmoniously, even though popular accounts emphasize conflicts and conspiracies. The global story of cultural change and interaction continues with the brutality of Christian Crusades and the great journeys of exploration and conquest, which diffused valuable knowledge, spices, and silks in all directions, while spreading destruction, suffering and death. Many written accounts of native peoples of the Americas, Africa, and Australia were produced by travelers and missionaries, such as the Franciscan priest Sahagún, who arrived in what is present-day Mexico in the early 1500s, learned the local Nahuatl language and made an invaluable contribution to Aztec historiography. While such accounts do not employ anthropological methodologies and are not claimed by most modern anthropologists as part of their direct scholarly genealogy, they provide an invaluable source of insight and background for interpreting and understanding contemporary anthropological data.

The classical object of anthropology has been for more than a century a deeper and more accurate, and more respectful understanding of "the other" and the worlds of others, in their varied social and experiential manifestations. From its inception, classical anthropological inquiry has sought to explore multiple social, political, and symbolic aspects of difference by seeking broad generalizations regarding human experience and commonalities among members of exotic communities and populations. As the founders of modern anthropology have shown (Malinowski, Evans-Pritchard, Douglas, Geertz, among others), even when the cultural others' schemes and practices for making sense of the world and the human condition seem utterly irrational to a Western observer, they are not less pragmatic or rational than the Westerner's elaborate biases and assumptions. Western scientific and medical education teaches young learners that the world operates according to the principles of Newton and Descartes in a manner that prioritizes the workings of the macroscopic physical and biological sciences and the notion of the neutral observer, making its pupils uneasy with the non-Western models of health, illness, and healing that employ nonphysical elements, which are difficult to measure and compare, such as one or multiple souls or spirits, or the ebb and flow of life force and healing energy through the bodies of participants as experienced during healing rituals.

A social science that aims to understand human behavior in its stunning diversity and complexity, contemporary anthropology draws on a distinct body of scholarly tradition and exploration of human cultures. The contemporary discipline of anthropology traces its roots only to the mid-nineteenth century, when scholars James George Frazer, Lewis Henry Morgan, and Edward Burnett Tylor produced extensive descriptive and analytical accounts of other people's religions, exploring the worldviews of small-scale and pre-literate societies, then labeled "primitive." Contemporary anthropology distinguishes itself from other humanities and social sciences by several characteristics, including an awareness and concern for the social context of practices (including history and politics), a cross-cultural and comparative perspective (drawing on a broad body of scholarship, theories, and data pertaining to different cultures), long-term ethnographic fieldwork using participant observation (the classic method of collecting anthropological data that involves the observer experientially and requires that the observer develops a rapport with the people and community being studied), reflexivity (examining one's own assumptions and biases and their impact on the study), holistic approach (recognizing that multiple aspects of culture interact and interrelate in any human experience or event), and a critical perspective (awareness of the role and dynamics of power and authority within and across all social boundaries).

The core concept of the American school of anthropology and a concept with a long tradition in the British and French school is *culture*, for which there are many possible definitions. John M. Janzen (2002:2–3) describes culture in his book *The Social Fabric of Health* as "creatively fashioned techniques, lifeways, social patterns, and deeply held convictions and assumptions in a community"; these are "stored and articulated in language"; they are learned; they change to contend with the limits of material conditions. A most remarkable human resource for adaptation through ideas, techniques, and organization and a quintessentially human achievement and adaptation, culture is learned, shared, integrated, patterned, and constantly changing in time and space. It has been demonstrated by leading proponents of symbolic theories of culture, such as Clifford Geertz and Mary Douglas, that cultures are not mere collections of expectations, behaviors, traditions, and social institutions, but complex *systems of meaning* embodied in and communicated through symbol systems. Languages everywhere are the key elements in the transmission of culture—symbolic systems of communication, actively engaged in shaping the cultural experiences of individuals and communities from birth to the end of life. People react to an environment as perceived and thought or understood, and most such experiences are mediated by language; some people fear black cats, many fear the word cancer, an envious gaze is said to bring illness and misfortune in Mediterranean villages. Different from values and norms, cultural *practices* are the lived aspects of culture, at work in everyday life, embedded in a web of shared meanings. From this perspective, which this writer endorses, to achieve a nuanced understanding of a social fact or phenomenon, such as alternative medicine, one must observe and reflect on the realm of everyday practices and explore the diverse social discourses accompanying them.

Medical anthropology, a newer subfield, focuses particularly on health-related beliefs and practices in their local cultural context. Medical anthropologists explore culturally situated ideas, norms, and practices related to health and illness, natural and supernatural. How is healing knowledge created, acquired, and legitimated in particular societies? How do behaviors, rituals, traditions, values, norms, and worldviews interact in regards to healing and health care? How do health, illness, and healing experiences vary with context? Health and healing are approached in a holistic and comparative manner: not as straightforward scientific facts but as cultural constructs, expressed symbolically through language, informed by particular historical, socioeconomic, and political circumstances.

Anthropologists draw on two centuries of detailed cross-cultural observations and a tremendous body of modern and contemporary scholarship in their efforts to understand how health and healing interrelate with other aspects, domains, and institutions within the cultural community in which they occur, and to recognize the value of indigenous knowledge and traditions, whether or not they can be substantiated with scientific proofs. A variety of theoretical approaches have risen to prominence since the 1960s, including, yet not limited to, the following (which are often interwoven in practice):

- biocultural: ecological anthropology, human variation, genomics, biosociality
- interpretive: hermeneutics, cultural classifications, and textuality of cultures
- anthropology of identity, ethnicity, and nationalism; conflict resolution

- anthropology of gender, contraception, reproduction, and birth
- anthropology of the body: the "three bodies" / the "mindful body"
- medical anthropology: ethnomedicine, ethnobotany, ethnopsychiatry
- medical ethnomusicology: cross-cultural views on music and healing
- critical medical anthropology: focus on power, authority, inequality
- phenomenological approaches to embodiment
- the anthropology of consciousness
- the sensory turn in anthropology

Healing Power and Agency

The ability to heal confers high status in all societies. Traditional healers are often born into families or lineages of healers and learn from a family member, who is also a healer. In many cases, folk healers have extraordinary birth circumstances or special signs associated with their birth. Sometimes they discover their calling through dreams or visions, severe illness, or a near-death experience. Experiencing a calling means that one must follow it or tragedy may befall the family. Folk healers learn by apprenticeship or experientially (also called "learning by doing"). The time spent in training may vary significantly, until the healer is ready to work on his or her own. In the absence of formal degrees or references, healers' success depends on their reputation and effectiveness. Many folk healers are herbalists and blend their own salves and tinctures. Some healers use divinatory rituals to diagnose illness, along with propitiatory rituals for ancestors and spirits; these may be accompanied by massage, drumming, chanting, or prayer.

The use of hallucinogenic plants for healing is not uncommon cross-culturally. For example, the mescaline-bearing cactus known as San Pedro is a popular hallucinogen used for therapeutic purposes for more than three thousand years in ancient Peru (Glass-Coffin 2010). When a patient takes San Pedro, it is in a ritual context, under close watch of the shaman, who monitors the amount ingested, looks out for the patient's well-being and interprets the visions, providing a context of meaning for the entire experience. In the case of the great medical traditions of India, China, and Greece-Arabia, there was and is the need for extensive formal study as well as apprenticeship, comparable to that of Western medical school. However, the practice of humoral medicine is generally considered to be empirical and individualized according to the patient's symptoms and characteristics. That is one confounding fact, from a Western perspective, that one may go to five different Ayurvedic or TCM physicians and come back with five different herbal blends or therapeutic recommendations. Due to the preference for single causes and single cures, a generic view of the patient, and the desire for standardization and risk management that characterize modern biomedicine, it is difficult for many of us Westerners to accept that all of those solutions may be equally valid and not suspect that some of the practitioners or all of them may be wrong. However, from an anthropological perspective, it is a common fact of healing in small-scale societies: neighboring tribes or two healers in the same rainforest community may use different parts of a plant for different purposes, with comparable success. From the perspective of ethnobotany, traditional plant-based medicines can contain dozens or hundreds of substances, which work in synergy. Some combinations may amplify or counteract one another's effects, or change the taste, or the color, and so on.

The power to heal is achieved in complex societies through formal and didactic education, which involves formal requirements, a lot of reading and writing, tests and exams. Just as complex and stratified societies have hierarchical religious orga-nizations, they also have strongly hierarchical healing systems. Whereas a patient and a folk healer usually share much of their language and worldview, the distance between biomedical doctors and their patients is vast and communication is impeded by terminology and social awkwardness, such as the hesitancy of patients to ask questions. The professionalization of disciplines (which has extended to osteopathy and chiropractic, as well as being increasingly common for other fields) has had the role of limiting entry into the health professions and protecting the income of those already in it. Because of third-party payment, rationing, and managed care, doctors are less able to devote a lot of time to a patient. There is also a trend (at least in the United States) of overfilling their schedules and letting patients wait in the waiting room for extended periods of time. Once in the office, a significant proportion of patients do not feel able to ask all the questions that they have or tell a full story. It is also true that patients in many cultures want to be helped with medicines and sometimes shots, rather than simply advice. The communication between patient and provider is a major component in the healing experience and a factor that affects compliance with recommendations as well as the likelihood that the patient will return. Several models of the doctor-patient relationship have been proposed. Veatch (1972) proposed the following:

- engineering model: patient directs his or her care and treatment; doctor assists
- priestly model: patient is passive, trusting, obedient; doctor has full authority
- contractual model: legal foundation, agreement of parties, mutual goals
- collegial model: trust between patient and doctor with equal effort

The model referred to as the priestly model is also commonly described as "pater-nalistic medicine" (from the Latin *pater*, meaning father). It is the kind of model that allows for the doctor to chastise the patient, exaggerate risks, or not communicate a terminal diagnosis. Some patients may prefer that kind of care, or at least expect it, whereas Westerners are increasingly encouraged to take responsibility for their own health, an attitude that is also very much part of the ethos of holistic medicine and CAM. Female patients born in countries where questioning a doctor's author-ity (or questioning him or her at all) is unacceptable tend to find it very difficult to participate actively in their care, as may patients with a language barrier. Also, in many cultures it is considered harmful to tell someone that he or she is dying (the Hmong for example consider this equivalent to a curse): this is something that medical doctors in the United States are expected to do, but patients from other cultures often do not want.

It is important to reflect on the importance of the sociological/anthropological notion of personal agency in the arena of health and healing: the power to act freely, even if it sometimes means resisting or challenging local norms and values. From the Foucaultian perspective of power as a capillary network, everyone has some forms of power at their disposal. This power, when combined with trust of the caregiver, can be harnessed as motivation and active participation in health care. From recent studies of CAM practitioners and modalities, as well as patients' motivations for seeking out and visiting CAM practitioners, it is evident that CAM practitioners tend to spend more time with the patients and more time listening to the patients' perceptions and experience of the illness. An initial homeopathic consult can last an hour or more, for example, a time when the patient is asked about every aspect of their well-being, from sleep habits, to cravings, to moods. Such individualized attention to detail and a greater willingness to listen to clients' concerns have contributed to the popularity of many alternative therapies, as biomedical practitioners often seek to elicit specific complaints (clearly identifiable as symptoms), dominate conversations, and expect unswerving obedience from patients. In *The Spirit Catches You and You Fall Down*, Anne Fadiman (1997:261) renders anthropologist and psychiatrist Arthur Kleinman's critique of the common term compliance, which he characterized as "lousy." In his view, for optimal outcome, a caregiver-patient relationship needs to be based on a model of mediation rather than one of coercion. Kleinman (1986, 1988) has been instrumental in developing the field of medical anthropology in the United States and globally, through his groundbreaking work on depression in China; his powerful exploration of the role of illness narratives in organizing, elucidating, and transforming experiences of sickness, pain, and disability; and his foundational, pioneering work on the anthropological study of social suffering.

What Are Cultural Constructions and Why Does It Matter to Health Care?

During the past three decades a substantial body of anthropological literature has shown that human biology, the construction of knowledge, and the relations of power within a social group are deeply interconnected domains. The creation and use of all medical knowledge is deeply enmeshed in cultural and historical circumstances and interactions, which are just as operative in the modern Western world as in other times and places (Foucault 1994 [1973]; Sontag 1990; Good 1994; Strathern 1996; Martin 1994, 2001, 2009). At one time, hysteria, onanism (i.e., masturbation), and drapetomania (the "disease" that caused slaves to run away, described in the mid-1800s by a Louisiana surgeon) were considered legitimate illness labels because they fit neatly with practical concerns, values, and inequities of a certain time and place. In some communist countries, those who spoke against iron-fisted regimes were sometimes declared mentally ill and put away in asylums. Now such diagnoses and therapies are viewed as pseudoscience (at best) or forms of exploitation, oppression, or abuse. When new diagnostic categories (such as alcoholism, PTSD, PMS, or pre-diabetes being a few recent additions) are created, legitimated, or sometimes deleted through overt and covert channels of power, it follows that policies, programs, and drugs are created and promoted to address the new diseases. Resources and blame are also redirected, along with the growing expectation that everyone affected take stock, reaching out for help and medication. Some newly designed categories and interventions can indeed improve the quality of life and avenues of support for many people, but the criteria and motivations of those involved in diagnosis and treatment are neither entirely clear-cut nor bias-free.

It should not be forgotten that the future success of new science enterprises such as *pharmacogenomics* (targeting drugs toward specific patient subpopulations based on their collected genetic information), depend on the diffusion across international boundaries of biocentric classification practices (such as the *DSM* of psychiatry), which are deeply embedded in modern capitalist economics and politics. These may be resisted or challenged at the local level by psychiatrists, psychoanalysts, and physicians who have "alternative" theoretical orientations or embrace local interpretations of illness. The Argentine psychoanalysts described by Lakoff (2005) deplore the North American emphasis on pharmaceutical management and the loss of speech-based therapy of a preceding era as dehumanizing to patients. In their view, the mechanistic brain-based approach of the new pharmaceutical psychiatry treats patients like animals and thus "erases 150 years of very rich history of psychiatry" (Lakoff 2005:64).

Locally and globally there are now new efforts and opportunities for protest and resistance, such as the Center for Cognitive Liberty and Ethics (CCLE), owner of the informative and provocative site titled cognitivliberty.org—an international organization founded by diverse group of activists, psychiatrists, academics, and artists. Group members share an urgent concern about the potential danger posed by pharmaceutical psychiatry and cognitive neurosciences and groups that do fit squarely with the norms and demands of current society and holders of power. Concerning the medicating of children diagnosed with ADHD (attention deficit and hyperactivity disorder), CCLE advocates for the right of parents (rather than school officials and teachers) to decide freely what measures to take and whether or how to "normalize" or modify their children's behaviors. Every person's focus could be improved with amphetamines, a biological fact that has lead to their use by college students, academics, and professionals as performance enhancers. Yet they do carry an array of serious risks, including the impaired growth in children and vascular damage, which may lead to sudden death. A range of alternative treatments exist for improving attention and reducing hyperactive behaviors, from the use of fish oils and DHA supplements to increasing the daily amount of exercise, changing the diet (eliminating refined sugar, carbohydrates, and artificial color), reducing the time spent in front of the television and electronic media, behavioral modification techniques, including biofeedback and meditation, essential oils (such as lavender), caffeine, or homeopathy (tarantula is such a remedy). The list of possibilities could go on and on. The production (and revision) of diagnostic categories that form the basis of professional expertise are periodically revised and redefined, alternately legitimated and challenged by ideologies, practices, and financial resources that inform them.

A Bird's Eye Overview of Core Concepts in Medical Anthropology

In modern capitalist settings, *health* is commonly described in materialist terms as the absence of disease, where *disease* is defined as a malfunction or disturbance, usually physical or biochemical in nature, which can be objectively identified based on externally established signs. From a holistic perspective, which acknowledges and includes nonbiological aspects of life—emotional, mental, social, and spiritual—health is best defined as a state of harmony, balance, and well-being. There are two "alternative" definitions of health that are in common usage, one negative (health as *absence* of disease) and the other positive (health as *presence* of well-being), and each definition generates a particular set of healthy and unhealthy people. One may have scientific evidence of physical disease but feel only negligible effects, thus be unhealthy by the biological definition but healthy by the other one (x-ray shows arthritis but it rarely hurts). Conversely, one may have no objective evidence of disease or malfunction, but experience pain—physical or mental—disturbed appetite, exhaustion, or other uncomfortable symptoms. This person may have good lab tests and no formal diagnosis, but nevertheless feel sick. Officially or physically, there is nothing detectably wrong, but the person is not feeling entirely well. From a holistic perspective, something is out of balance: there is disharmony. The roots of this suffering could be interpreted as social, emotional, or supernatural, depending on one's cultural and personal beliefs. Diverse healing traditions (such as shamanism, acupuncture, faith healing, etc.) each have ways of addressing the discomfort and rebalancing physical and nonphysical aspects of a person to restore health and promote long-term well-being.

It is valuable to compare the two definitions of health with two similar definitions of beauty, to explore the consequences of definitions on the way we carve out reality. If we define beauty as absence of blemishes or flaws, we have one set of beautiful things (which depends of course on how we define the word blemish or flaw). Thus, a woman with freckles or a prominent mole or a scar, could, according to some judgments, be excluded on that basis from the "beautiful" set of people. However, if beauty is defined in positive terms, as harmonious, balanced, or pleasant appearance, those blemishes may matter less. In fact, according to some cultural traditions, such features may enhance the beauty of the person or object involved. In Japan, a small crack in a lovely old piece of porcelain only makes it more beautiful and desirable. This is not unlike the European concept of *patina*, which refers to gentle signs of wear on a valuable object, thus signs of past life and enjoyment. The ways in which we define the set plays a big role in people's perceptions and decisions about what belongs and what does not. Much like beauty, health is not a hard fact of life, but a personal judgment and a subjective experience, in the mind of the beholder. How do persons and communities decide who is healthy and who is sick? What are criteria for inclusion and exclusion? What are the solutions?

Homeopath David Owen (2007:3) writes that "how we understand the relationship between the substance and energy of life determines the model we use to describe health." He describes no less than five models of health, noting that the way the practitioner describes health and defines illness determines his or her approach to treatment and the prescribing methodology. The *pathogenic* model looks at an external cause, or *aetiology*. The *biological* model focuses on symptoms, recognizing that a single cause may produce different effects in different systems. In his usage of the term, the *holistic* model recognizes that many aspects of patient and environment are involved, connected through mutual feedback, and that illness may be necessary in order to effect a needed change in the environment or the person. The *holographic* model suggests that symptoms that may happen in different areas of the body or the person; any part or symptom will reflect the whole picture and (if known fully) can express "the essence of the patient." Finally, the *relational* model highlights the role of the context of symptoms and the patient's relationships, including the relationship with the healer; in the case of a homeopathic practitioner, Owen states that the homeopath's own sensation, reflections and awareness may provide valuable intuitive information.

Sometimes used interchangeably in popular culture, disease and illness represent two very different notions in medical sociology and anthropology. Reflecting the methods and values of science and the goal of objective assessment, the term *disease* usually points to a biological malfunction, pathology or a degenerative process, identified based on externally established signs, through clinical diagnosis or technological media, usually by a medical professional. The term *illness* describes the subjective experience of impaired functioning from the perspective of the sufferer, whether or not there is evidence or confirmation of a disease process. Illnesses represent the personal and social experience of malfunction or discomfort in particular cultural contexts. Thus, two people with osteoarthritis of the knee or the wrist may have the same disease but vastly different illness experiences depending on particular demographics and socioeconomics: age and gender, income and insurance, work and family obligations and support networks, ability to fill needed drug prescriptions, and accessibility of resources for nonbiomedical care, which may

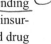

prevent further deterioration, such as regular exercise, supplements, or alternative therapies. Education, personality, interpretations about the causes and meanings of pain or illness, social stigma, and spiritual beliefs also affect how one responds to discomfort, physical limitations, and disability, or how people cope with the impact of illness. Politics play a major role as well: whether the government mandates or covers certain services, treatments, or sick leave, or whether certain groups and minorities are identified as "at risk" and targeted in various ways for education or treatment. All of these dimensions are part of the cultural context of illness and suffering, not just the localized phenomenon that scientists and clinicians commonly call disease.

Curing or Healing?

Healing is a therapeutic process or action that addresses the whole suffering person and the illness, rather than just a specific body part or a particular problem, thus including emotional, mental, social, and spiritual needs and concerns in the treatment plan. Healing aims at bringing about improvement in various areas of experience and promoting overall well-being, even if (or when) a cure is uncertain or unlikely. *Curing* refers to a narrower and more pragmatic approach, which has the goal of removing a particular problem completely and permanently, whether that may be a disease, social or spiritual disorder, mental or emotional dysfunction, or a spell. Whereas curing aims at eliminating specific conditions or harm, healing seeks to reestablish harmony and provide relief physically, emotionally, mentally, and socially, but it may mean living through illness or living with illness, even when a cure may not be achievable. Healing aims to restore wellness or balance to the person as whole, including the social fabric unraveled by loss, conflict or distress, not just the individual body or part afflicted with misfortune or disease. In traditional settings, the family and community are usually involved in healing experiences. In practice, healing and curing are not mutually exclusive or easily distinguishable. They can intertwine, overlap, or even be one and the same process.

There are many interpretations of the difference between curing and healing, in lay and scholarly terms. UK practitioner and activist Patrick Quanten (2002), who renounced his medical license in 2001 to devote himself exclusively to complementary therapies, provides an impassioned, persuasive, tendentious critique of biomedical curing and the healing/curing contrast on his *Active Health* website. Quanten argues that the notion of "cure" has been hijacked by the medical establishment and drug manufactures, which emphasize the elimination or destruction of external forces of illness (such as germs) for the purpose of restoration of well-being. In contrast, 'healing is about 'making whole,'' Quanten observes—there is no enemy, nothing to be destroyed, and the state of wholeness achieved by healing does not need to be the same as the original state of being.

Anthropologists Andrew Strathern and Pamela Stewart (1999) have provided a detailed ethnographic exploration of healing and curing from a medical anthropology perspective, drawing richly on their own fieldwork with native groups in the Mount Hagen area of New Guinea. Strathern and Stewart (1999:55) distinguish Melpa curers, who use spells to correct physical problems, from local healers who address illness caused "by immoral or improper actions." Definite or absolute distinctions regarding whether a healing practice or experience constitutes curing or healing, or whether it is "holistic" are surprisingly difficult to apply cross-culturally, because they are complicated by the observer's notions of where and how the realms of the mental, emotional and physical are bounded, as well as the spatial, relational and spiritual boundaries of the self, which are determined by culture. In discussing Japanese *Kanpo* (or *Kampo*), the medical system brought to Japan from China in the sixth century, now commonly blended with cosmopolitan or Western medicine, Strathern and Stewart observed that Margaret Lock's (1980) and Emiko Ohnuki-Tierney's (1984) interpretations differed significantly, particularly regarding the notion of *ki*. The energy, also known as *qi* or *chi* in East Asian traditions, is widely referenced by contemporary practitioners of CAM and integrative medicine, being commonly equated with spirit or mind. Lock's ethnographic analysis states that *ki* is equivalent to the flux of emotions, whereas Ohnuki-Tierney insists that *ki* does not pertain to the domain of psychology, but rather physiology. She has coined the term *physiomorphism* to describe how various factors such as chill winds and inborn constitutions (involving nerves and blood types that correlate with the acidity or alkalinity of foods) contribute to bodily imbalance. It is telling, indeed, that two leading scholars of health and healing have interpreted *ki* so differently (Strathern and Stewart 1999:24).

The history and social context of medical notions and ideas about etiology or the interplay of forces that shape health and sickness are unique to every experiential and cultural setting. Most life experience is mediated through our bodies and deeply embedded in cultural context. As explored in subsequent chapters, illness and healing cannot be equated with the generic and sequential listings of symptoms or stages described in medical textbooks and diagnostic manuals, which are the result of political and administrative decisions, as well as history. Illness and healing are enmeshed in the vivid social fabric of everyday lives, manifested through sensory engagements uniquely formed in each cultural setting, colored by personal memory and experience, then given meaning through the lenses of past and present relationships, interactions and events, both collective and personal.

Whereas in Western terms "mind-body healing" is by default considered holistic because it addresses mind *and* body, in Japan these boundaries are clearly not the same, nor firmly drawn, while in small scale societies the social dimension is fundamental. Fluctuations of *ki* or uncontrolled emotions can cause a wide range of discomforts, threatening the linkages of life-force between body, environment, and the social world, as well as proper functioning within the body. It is significant to recall that according to Japanese tradition and folk beliefs, the life-soul or vital essence of the self resides in the stomach area rather than the head, heart, or mind as it does in Western societies. From this perspective, the socially commendable practice of *harakiri,* the traditional form of suicide of Samurai warriors of medieval Japan, is recognizable as a last-resort "cure" for dishonor: releasing the self by slashing open the abdomen. But it can also be construed as a form of healing, following Strathern and Stewart's interpretation: redressing the social imbalance and disruption created by wrongful or immoral action. This act of curing or healing causes the death of the body, as it mends the social self.

Biomedicine and Traditional Medicine

Biomedical sciences employ a mechanical model of the human body and tend to treat each organ and each person in isolation from others, emphasizing individual *etiology* (causation) and responsibility (. . . or blame). Biomedicine is also characterized by the search for the "magic bullet": the *one* treatment, drug or chemical factor that treats or cures the disease. In contrast, traditional or folk models of health and healing tend to look at illness as resulting from a combination of *multiple* natural and supernatural causes, requiring a combination of therapies or ingredients to achieve a cure. According to such models, healing rituals, prayers, herbal medicines, and biomedical care can all be used in concert to restore harmony with natural, social, and spirit worlds in order to achieve improvement or recovery. The *sociological model of illness* emphasizes the role of sociopolitical factors over individual ones; critical medical sociology and anthropology focus particularly on power and inequality as key factors in morbidity and mortality patterns. Disease patterns reflect socioeconomic distinctions.

An important finding of anthropological and sociological scholarship is that, like illness, normality is shaped by cultural forces, needs, and expectations. While all societies recognize certain behaviors as undesirable or disruptive, in Western societies, the biomedical model is applied frequently to such behaviors: they are considered to be medical problems with medical solutions. Realms of human experience previously considered part of the everyday life and outside the domain of biomedicine are brought under the surveillance and control of medical professionals as forms of sickness or deviance. Some examples include alcoholism, birth, infertility, oppositional defiant disorder, and pre-diabetes. A combination of the tyranny of the normal and the popular quest for eternal youth that plagues modern capitalist societies is recognizable when a woman with very small breasts is described by surgeons as having "micromastia," along with feelings of stress and inadequacy, and offered breast surgery, or a woman entering menopause as having a hormone deficiency disease and prescribed hormone replacement therapy, which carries increased risk of strokes and some cancers. The complex social phenomenon of providing official medical labels and medical solutions to things previously considered part of normal life experience has been called *medicalization* and is a major topic in contemporary medical sociology and anthropology (Conrad 2007; Weitz 2009; Davis-Floyd 2004; Horwitz 2002; Lock 1995). Such normative determinations of function or appearance are often accompanied by expensive medical solutions for "problems" that were previously simply considered part of the normal spectrum of life experiences, in this case, women's experiences. Concomitant with medicalization, there have been strong initiatives toward de-medicalization, such as the natural and home birth movements and other so-called alternative health movements.

Biomedicine strongly emphasizes the idea of normal functioning, either as an aim of therapeutic actions or as a goal of preventive efforts. "Target" ranges of vital parameters and bodily substances (such as weight, height, red blood cells, glucose, cholesterol, etc.) are considered desirable or ideal on the basis of large-scale biostatistical calculations. Numbers for such biological measurements tend to fall along a statistical curve called the normal distribution or "the bell curve," with most people somewhere in the middle of the bell, and numbers of people declining toward the left and right edges. The term "tyranny of the normal" has been used critically to describe an overemphasis on normality that leads to social stigma or excessive interference with the minds and bodies of people who do not meet cultural criteria of normality. This cultural tyranny (or social pressure) is what leads some expectant parents to abort a fetus diagnosed with dwarfism, to avoid the social and medical consequences of such a condition. But this kind of decision has incited protests from communities of "little people" who fear that the often meaningful and productive existence of such persons (documented on Earth since the dawn of mankind) may be now greatly threatened with the advent of prenatal screening technologies, which assist parents in the quest for the perfect offspring. Analogously, any child who is very small for his or her age may be targeted for intervention in a biomedical system and be given a diagnosis and considered a risk (insurance has at times been denied to such children in the United States) and offered therapies (that may have serious side-effects), even though that child may be functioning well otherwise.

Deviance from the norm (in behavior, appearance, or any other way) is often frowned on cross-culturally. In some cases it may be rewarded, but more often it is feared. For example, in the parts of Central and Southern Europe and the Middle East, where most people's hair and eyes are dark, green or blue eyes are said to give the "evil eye" or bring bad luck. Red hair, which is also unusual, being caused by a recessive gene, has been associated with witchcraft. In various African countries, albino children and adults have been recently kidnapped and killed for their bodies, fragments of which are employed by some sorcerers for their powerful magic; retreats and shelters have been created to try to protect survivors from harm. Biomedically, deviance from the norm is commonly targeted with corrective efforts: typically drugs, surgery, or sometimes dietary and lifestyle management. Labeling of illness occurs through a mix of scientific and political mechanisms that are not value free, involving complex interactions of cultural knowledge, power, and authority. The creation of new illness labels can bring prestige or financial rewards, particularly when associated with new methods of diagnosis of therapy. The rise of ADHD treatment in North America is an example of this nexus: after the introduction of Ritalin in the second half of the twentieth century the popularity of this diagnosis and its drug therapy skyrocketed, with millions of prescriptions of psychotropic drugs being used annually by North American boys. Despite great technological and economic progress in modern capitalism, the lines between physical, mental, and social illness may be just as blurred in the West as in small-scale societies.

Whereas altered states of consciousness (ASCs) are commonly considered deviant according to Western ideals of mental clarity, rationality, and control, they are natural states and propensities of the human brain. Humans have experienced such states since the dawn of humankind and in small-scale societies they are often used in the context of healing rituals. ASCs can be induced naturally or using processed substances, intentionally or unintentionally. Dance and other forms of repetitive body movement, drumming and other forms of rhythmic sound, rhythmic breathing, excessive heat, hunger, solitude and isolation, meditation, flashing lights, and strong emotions (love, fear, shock) can all induce ASCs. Some social groups and traditional healers use plant substances like tobacco, peyote, or mushrooms. In the United States and Mexico, the use of certain psychoactive plants is legal only in a religious or ritual setting.

Westerners commonly turn to pharma drugs, alcohol, and tobacco to reduce pain or induce pleasurable states; in contrast to traditional drug use, these experiences are most commonly sought without the close supervision, monitoring, and guidance of experienced healers. At the beginning of this new millennium, coffee seems to be the psychoactive substance of choice throughout much of the world, followed by alcohol and tobacco products, antidepressants, and ADHD medications. The latter two are becoming popular enhancement drugs. In some societies mental conditions currently stigmatized in the modern West, such as schizophrenia or epilepsy, may indicate that someone is destined to become a healer and help others. Many folk healers come from families of healers and have to apprentice with an experienced healer to become one. Most folk healers experience a calling: a dream, a vision, severe illness, or a near-death experience, which tells them that they have to follow a healing path. Disobeying it can lead to misfortune.

The term *ethnomedicine* is broadly used in anthropology to refer to local healing traditions and practices within a cultural context. Every band or tribe or village in the world has ethnomedical knowledge. It is fairly easy for a non-native observer to apprehend that "folk healing" methods are embedded in the history of the community and a particular culture area, and that practices reflect a group's relationship with the natural environment, its interaction with the invisible worlds of spirits and ancestors, and its social experiences, past and present. But whereas anthropologists initially described only local healing traditions distinct from contemporary Western medicine as ethnomedical traditions, it has become accepted that *biomedicine itself is a type of ethnomedicine*: the product of particular history of ideas, distinctive practices of knowledge creation, and varied socioeconomic-political influences. These influences are uniquely and inextricably tied to the cultural history of Western Europe, the Enlightenment tradition of mind-body separation, the subsequent rise of industrialism and capitalism, and most recently, to the contemporary forces of information technology, biotechnology, and globalization. As all ethnomedical traditions are marked and shaped by their origins, histories, and the steady flux of modern cultural exchange, so is biomedicine.

Health and healing traditions outside biomedicine tend to emphasize ideas of balance and harmony and personal well-being, rather than standards and norms of functionality. Traditional or folk medicine, as it is often called, is commonly a blend of naturalistic and personalistic beliefs and practices, such as herbalism or humoralism, and rituals related to ancestors, spirits of nature, or the divine. Most contemporary environments are characterized by various degrees of *medical pluralism*: the presence of multiple medical systems or traditions; patients usually combine or try to take advantage of a variety of methods, starting with the most accessible (such as home care and local healers) and, depending on the seriousness of the problem, going on to more expensive and invasive techniques, like biomedicine. The spirit or supernatural world and its effects on one's well-being are as real for some cultures as the world of germs (or pop stars) is for ours.

An often unintended effect of positive expectation in therapeutic encounters, the *placebo effect* plays a powerful role in all healing experiences, including biomedical encounters. In modern clinical trials, it helps elucidate the impact of new drugs and procedures, which are compared to the effects of "sugar pill" placebos and the effects of no intervention. While being a basic and universal phenomenon, it is challenging to define, in part because of its paradoxical nature: feeling better from taking a sugar pill looks like getting something from nothing and may even seem like fraud in an evidence- and market-driven society. But that "nothing" of the placebo is far from nothing at all: it is the impact of anticipation, meaning, and the cultural context of healing. Anthropologist Daniel Moerman (2000:52) defined placebo effects as "desirable psychological and physiological effects of meaning in the treatment of illness." It has been amply shown to play a role in all healing encounters and to be a tremendous ally in traditional healing practices, especially ritual and religious healing, where symbols (which may be words, gestures, images, or objects) often constitute key therapeutic tools. It seems unfair and unfortunate that this is often equated with deceit in biomedical circles. A powerful healing resource, the placebo effect does not account for all nonbiomedical healing, some of which involves the use of medicines, manipulation and other specific remedies. Its working is not an indication that symptoms are "fake" or "only in someone's head," that the person is mentally unhealthy or a hypochondriac (all of which are common popular misconceptions of placebos). It is a genuine and powerful healing force in its own right, richly and creatively employed in local healing practices worldwide.

Many traditional treatments and rituals manipulate the human body, as well as the human mind to achieve relief from physical, mental, and social distress. Respected healers tend to have abundant knowledge of their environments and the social and spiritual worlds of their patients, which they usually share and know intimately, thus practicing healing methods that can address a broader range of patient needs and may be characterized as holistic. Biomedicine emphasizes the mechanical aspects of the human body, preferring mono-causal explanations, "magic bullet" cures, and broad generalizations. It often promotes invasive, expensive, high-tech approaches, administered generically and individually, rather than at the level of a social group. Biomedical practitioners are typically more distanced from their patients than traditional healers, due to high socioeconomic status and highly specialized knowledge. Pharmaceutical drugs are extensively (and expensively) researched, highly processed and concentrated, and aggressively marketed to physicians and the general public. In many cases, biomedical drugs aim to suppress symptoms (pain, rashes, etc.) without attempting to address the social or psychological suffering that accompanies them. They commonly contain one or few active ingredients. In contrast, traditional medicines are closer to their natural form and often contain a multitude of ingredients, which work in concert with one another, amplifying or reducing each other's effects. It is more difficult to consume a deadly overdose on traditional medicines, but many have powerful effects and should be used with caution, preferably under the supervision of a herbalist or traditional healer.

As popularized in the Western world today, "natural healing" blends various sources of traditional and scientific knowledge, emphasizing a gentle approach: seeking harmony with nature through remedies that are minimally processed and working with the body-soul-mind as a whole to restore balance within and without. In their original (local) versions, traditional healing practices have not always been "gentle," sometimes involving bitter or toxic herbal medicines and potions, vomiting, purging, animal sacrifices, and a wide range of physical and mental discomforts to drive out illness or bad spirits. But in the modern marketplace of alternatives to biomedicine, there has been a selective pressure toward gentler forms of traditional healing, which most modern consumers of healing alternatives seek and prefer.

The "gentle" stereotype is often contrasted with the aggressiveness of modern scientific medicine, which encourages doctors to fight disease as the evil enemy. This is aptly illustrated by the case of a pediatric oncologist who refuses to stop chemotherapy treatment even when death is imminent, or the ob-gyn doctor who pressures a laboring woman into having a C-section because the end of his or her shift is approaching, or his/her concern with being sued. Such modern physicians embody modern medicine's desire to control nature and timing, a view that nature should not be allowed to take its course or lead the way, and that doing something is better than doing nothing. Disease is seen as the ultimate villain. For health professionals who share this aggressive and confrontational worldview, it is better to keep fighting a losing battle than to let sickness "win," no matter what the human emotional toll may be for patients or their families. In this heroic view, nature verges on chaos and humans are its conquerors. This feature of "allopathic medicine" is heir to the "heroic medicine" that preceded it in the eighteenth and nineteenth centuries, when early Western physicians and surgeons employed abrasive treatments such as bleeding and purging to ward off disease. Many of the healing currents that emerged in the nineteenth century (such as homeopathy and Christian Science) defined themselves in contrast to this aggressive ethos reminiscent of colonial conquest. Not surprisingly, such healing modalities, which questioned the authoritative and paternalistic approach to healing, turned out to have a particular appeal to women and minorities. The ethos of conquest contrasts also with animistic worldviews that tend to characterize small-scale societies with kin-based and household-based social organization. There the relationship with nature is perceived and represented as an intimate one: a bond of kinship. Even illness and death are a part of the natural and supernatural order.

As child-bearers, women are everywhere involved in nurturing and caring, as expressed in Florence Nightingale's famous statement that "every woman is a nurse." But captured in this same statement is the marginalization and sometimes exclusion of women from the roles and accounts of healing in Western societies, which has been a recurrent pattern. As European medicine developed during the middle ages under close scrutiny from Christian religious authorities, the activities of women who deviated from social expectations were viewed with suspicion. Herbalists and wise-women (including some visionary nuns and ascetics) who were skilled in healing have at various times been perceived by clergy and male doctors as a threat to tradition and their own authority, some being persecuted as witches. The fairytale stereotype of the witch reveals her as the cultural construction that she is, embodying the polar opposite of the social ideal of womanhood in Medieval Europe. The witch lives entirely alone and shirks company, sometimes by going deep into the forest, without fear; she has a sickly colored complexion, sallow or green, an enormous warty nose, and unkempt hair, sometimes unnaturally red, a symbol of sexuality and sin; she is old, dirty and ill-tempered, fervent despiser and incorrigible eater of children, riding her broom (and thus perverting a symbol of domesticity) like a horse (another not-to-be missed sexual connotation). Her powers are threatening, self-serving, and toxic, like her herbal concoctions, which she makes by boiling suspicious and secret ingredients in a big black cauldron. She is selfish and moody and keeps very odd pets. This character is the ultimate contrast with the ideal Christian woman: married, subservient, humble, nurturing, caring, fertile, industrious woman, who uses the broom to clean; tames her hair; depends on God, clergy, and her husband for answers; and sleeps at night, bearing no secrets or secret life.

Thus someone who is socially marginal and does not meet social expectations for reciprocity (sharing and exchange) becomes a scapegoat, in a process that releases and externalizes social tensions about property and control. Anthropologists have observed that witchcraft beliefs are more common in societies where there is accumulation of private property, particularly agricultural societies, with a notion of limited good (limited resources that must be divided up, so that if one person gets more, another one inevitably gets less), whereas hunters and gatherers are less likely to be concerned with witchcraft. In African societies witches can be men or women and are commonly believed to have an inner essence that enables them to cause harm to others, even unconsciously. But women are more commonly accused than men and accusations are likely to happen among co-wives in a polygynous marriage, if and when their fortunes seem to markedly differ. A woman who seems particularly successful in some way that is not traditionally feminine can cause envy and suspicion. When misfortune occurs, witch hunters use divination to identify a particular person or relationship as the culprit. The person must confess, reparations may be required, or she or he may be expelled from the community, temporarily or permanently. Not adequately participating in social exchange or exhibiting illegitimate powers can lead to an accusation of witchcraft. In societies where witchcraft beliefs are functioning as an explanatory system, most illness and misfortune can be traced to such a cause, even if a natural cause is recognized as well.

The role of women as healers and caregivers for the sick is well documented worldwide, but their participation in medicine was repeatedly undermined, discouraged, and limited in Western societies, where until recently the healing profession has been uniformly dominated by white males, even in the arena of birthing. Women were extremely active in the popular sector of health care and in eighteenth-century America many worked as lay doctors, often sharing a practice with their husbands. The Popular Health Movement in the 1830s and 1840s merged the interests of women and the working classes in the United States and emphasized preventive care and hygiene in the public or official arena. Midwives are becoming increasingly popular, after a long period of marginalization by the AMA. Among alternative medicine users today, women have been and continue to be a majority, and their participation as practitioners of CAM continues to grow, although they face additional challenges establishing themselves professionally because of family demands.

Influential scholars Emily Martin (2001), Gail Kligman (1998), Margaret Lock (1995), and others have shown that women's biosocial lives have been subject to more negative labeling and regulation under medical regimes (in medical literature and clinical practice) than men's bodies, which are often taken to represent the standard of normal biology. In this vein, monthly ovulation and bleeding have been portrayed as destructive processes and hormone fluctuations as undesirable, while symptoms of certain common ailments (like heart disease or chronic pain) may be overlooked or downplayed, if they differ significantly from the men's. Women's bodies are the "other" of men's bodies and their functioning is therefore "alternative" to men's. Not coincidentally, women have been at the forefront of folk and home-based healing traditions and have been shown to be more frequent users and supporters of alternative and complementary approaches, in the United States and elsewhere.

Plural Healing in the Global Age: Intersections of Meaning and Power

Medical pluralism—the coexistence of multiple healing options, methods or systems—is characteristic of most non-Western settings today. In Western nations healing alternatives have reappeared in force after having faded from the public eye for many decades (particularly in the United States), and are gradually being co-opted into the mainstream under the gloss of CAM. These burgeoning new markets of services and products in which the poorest may not be able to fully partake are often interpreted as an expression of public disenchantment with the humanistic shortcomings of scientific medicine. However, among immigrants and refugees, as well as throughout the so-called developing world, a strategic blending of therapies is usually encountered. The patterns of care-seeking often follow a logical sequence, described by the notion of "hierarchies of resort," developed by Lola Romanucci-Ross (1969) and based on her fieldwork in Melanesia. People commonly rely on older medical systems and local healing traditions *before* seeking biomedical treatment, as practices of "first resort." Local healers may incorporate various biomedical concepts and tools into their own healing work, and may even refer their patients for biomedical care, if needed. Frequently, our concept of "alternative healing" has no local equivalent. From this latter perspective, scientific medicine could indeed be called *alternative*. In settings where there are classical or indigenous healing traditions being practiced, typically more affordable and accessible, modern scientific medicine is generally not the patient's first choice, but the "last resort."

Although real-world practitioners of healing do not tend to fit neatly into dualistic frameworks, anthropologists recognize two broad types of illnesses and healing approaches, based on the classic typology proposed decades ago by Foster and Anderson (1978). *Naturalistic explanations* emphasize the physical body and the environment as causative and therapeutic agents: injuries, deterioration, blockage, exertion, seasonal changes, temperature extremes, imbalances of bodily fluids, diet, poisons, germs, and so on. In contrast, *personalistic explanations* prioritize the role of social and supernatural factors, from interpersonal conflict, emotions (particularly anger, jealousy, and envy), damage to the soul or loss of soul, intrusion of foreign objects into the body by magical means, spirit aggression, witchcraft and sorcery, or punitive action by ancestors, spirits, or divine entities. Commonly, naturalistic explanations point to unintentional harm, whereas personalistic explanations tend to point to intentional harm. Among the "great medical traditions" that have ample written records and a distinct historical continuity going back thousands of years, such as India's Ayurveda, TCM, classical Greek and Greco-Roman medicine, and Unani Tibb, the Greco-Arabic tradition, the emphasis tends to be placed on naturalistic explanations. Esteemed practitioners of these influential medical systems are predominantly empirical, pragmatic, reasoned, and flexible in their application of diagnostic methods and therapies, providing individualized treatment based on extensive formal knowledge and clinical experience. Based on a thorough evaluation of the patient, it is common that food, herbs, and physical manipulation are provided as remedies for illness, with the intent of restoring a state of balance to the individual. Still, traditional healers tend to resort to a blend of naturalistic and personalistic explanations and remedies. Foods, herbs, and rituals are interwoven to achieve maximum efficacy. This is the case with *susto*, a fright illness common in Latin America, which involves potentially life-threatening soul loss. It may be triggered by a naturalistic event, such as tripping on a rock, or by a personalistic one, such as a nighttime encounter with a ghost or an upsetting social event. The usual cure is a series of healing rituals that begin with Catholic prayer, administered by a local *curandero* in the presence of family and friends. Sometimes an egg or herbs may be rubbed over the patient's body to neutralize the illness and offerings made to the spirit that has captured the patient's soul. The patient may be sprayed with alcohol from the healer's mouth, massaged vigorously, or made to sweat. In mild cases of *susto,* a medicinal tea made of herbs (such as marijuana) may suffice as a cure (O'Neil 2006).

The distinction between the natural and the supernatural is often made in Western cultures. It has been widely used in cultural anthropology, as well, in the definition of religion. However, Morton Klass (1995) points out that such a definition reflects an ethnocentric and scientific bias: the researcher imposes preexisting categories on cultural practices he or she observes, but the native people performing rituals or carrying out traditional practices do not necessarily make the same distinctions. During his fieldwork with East Indian peasants in Trinidad, Klass (1995:28–9) realized that a guardian spirit of the field was no less "natural" to a farmer making a sacrificial offering than the absentee landlord to whom the farmer must pay part of the harvest as rent: the farmer had never met either one of them. Similarly, in healing contexts, it can be argued that an afflicting spirit is no less real or natural from the perspective of an indigenous healer than a virus or a mutation may be to a Western health professional. Both are experienced as uncontestable realities or facts. Thus, anthropologically speaking, the notion of *fact* has two separate meanings: from an outsider perspective, such as that of an external observer (called *etic* in classical anthropology), it refers to a true or objective reality, which presumably exists; from an insider point of view (a native or indigenous perspective, called *emic* in anthropology) "it refers to that which, in a given human society, is understood to be reality" (Klass 1995:50). People know the cultural facts of their own culture, which they acquire from birth through an embodied experience.

Anthropologists found that the notion of belief, while greatly emphasized in Western societies and traditions, tends to be secondary to practice(s) in traditional settings, where what a Western observer may perceive as extraordinary or evidence of supernatural beliefs is simply an everyday experience or awareness by local standards. It is not what one believes that matters most, but what one does: the need to uphold traditional practices (rituals and taboos) in relation to spirits, people, and the surrounding environment is a common and natural reality of life. In their efforts to explain the world, or the source of one's illness, people rarely resort to a single source or type of explanation outside biomedical settings. Most often, etiologies and therapies combine the natural and the supernatural, considering multiple causes and multiple remedies. A Romanian grandmother may rub the wrist while chanting the Lord's Prayer, before and after uttering in hushed voice a traditional spell for removing evil-eye magic, while at the same time administering hot herbal teas or possibly other remedies, such as a hot foot bath and a dose of aspirin or acetaminophen, thus covering all bases.

In contemporary Western settings, there are definite similarities between CAM integrative approaches and New Age syncretism: they both rely on a blending of traditions, being concomitantly pluralistic and universalizing; they both challenge monistic and orthodox explanations and authority; and they have both been spurred and facilitated significantly by globalization and the new electronic media, alongside other forms of cultural *bricolage*.

Writing about contemporary religious perspectives, Morton Klass (1995) offered the moniker "post-rationalists" to describe persons who deny the existence of a single source of higher knowledge, having become dissatisfied with both science and religious fundamentalism, yet still finding some value in both traditions. To them, science does not have all the answers and it is vulnerable to bias and error, just like other human endeavors. At the same time, no religious tradition or text is considered totally without merit, as they all may provide valuable insights and contain valuable kernels of truth. Unity and universalism are thus touchstones of the post-rationalist perspective, which upholds that "*nothing* is ever *completely* wrong" (Klass 1995:162).

Klass's post-rationalism is cousin to postmodernism, the theoretical perspective that marked a powerful reflective turn in the social sciences. Postmodernists reject claims to objective truth by a neutral observer with the recognition that there is great diversity and inherent bias in individual experiences, which are not and cannot be subsumed in totalizing meta-narratives. In this view, no value-free and culture-free endeavor or authority exists that can legitimize only one source of knowledge above all others. In the social sciences this has also been experienced as a "crisis of representation" that points to the limitations set on us by our own labels and categories of understanding. Can we accurately represent other people's worlds or experiences if all we have is our own preexisting labels and frameworks, deeply imprinted through socialization, beginning from birth? These questions lie at the heart of contemporary anthropological scholarship. Similarly, post-rationalism holds that there is no one "Truth," but many "truths," so there is an interest in sharing perspectives and experiences among those who come from different backgrounds. Convinced that there is no single answer to the problems our planet faces, post-rationalists are "prepared to listen to all suggestions" and believe "that the solution will require the triumph of universalism." Klass wrote:

> Post-rationalists are therefore free to move without guilt from faith to faith, to accept any elements of the faiths of their parents, or even of science, without feeling any necessity to accept anything else or to worry about mutual exclusivity of beliefs. What is significant, therefore, is not the differences between all these post-rationalists, as I have labeled them, but what they have in common: their acceptance of one another—not necessarily of one another's beliefs or interests but of their common quest for meaning and comfort in a world where anything is possibly true and nothing can be known for certain. (1995:162)

It is valuable to recognize how closely Klass's perspective connects with a very recent trend in integrative medicine, exemplified by Gerard C. Bodeker's (2008) pioneering efforts, which integrate global public health initiatives, traditional knowledge and methods for controlling and managing illness (including malaria, HIV, skin diseases), and the efforts, wisdom and skills of local health practitioners and refugees in East and Southeast Asia. Australian-born and Harvard-trained in epidemiology, Bodeker teaches at University of Oxford Medical School and Columbia's Mailman School of Public Health, where he is affiliated with The Rosenthal Center for Complementary and Alternative Medicine, and collaborates with the World Health Organization and other international bodies to bring creative and integrative solutions to global public health crises. Among Bodeker's accomplishments are the creation of the Global Initiative for Traditional Systems (GIFTS) of Health (giftsofhealth.org) and WHO-affiliated Research Initiative on Traditional Anti-malarial Methods (RITAM), which he co-founded. He is an authority of medicinal plants, and is also actively involved in global conservation efforts. While biomedicine and epidemiology emerged from radically different worldviews and methodologies than indigenous ethnobotanical traditions, a joining of such diverse efforts is currently justified by a deep recognition that there is no single answer and that people with profoundly different perspectives on illness and healing need to come together for common goals.

Current Practice: Helminths Return as Promising New Drugs

If health is construed environmentally, as a balanced symbiotic relationship that benefits both an organism and its environment, many modern practices are decidedly unhealthy. Humans' extended global wars on germs and parasites have pitted individuals against their natural environments, seeking to establish human dominance through elimination of all potentially invasive organisms known to cause sickness. The possibility that pests and parasites had an instrumental role in human well-being was rarely (or never) considered until recently. In 1989 David Strachan noted that children born into small families were more prone to hay fever, suggesting that early exposure to infectious agents may prevent allergic rhinitis (Strachan 1989). Thus, the hygiene hypothesis was born, stating that decreased exposure to infectious agents early in life increases susceptibility to allergy and perhaps autoimmune diseases by limiting immune system development (Kersiek 2008). From an ecological perspective, the hygiene hypothesis and the rehabilitation of microbes provide an alternative model of human-ecosystem interaction, which challenges older biomedical models of health and disease. Can a person with parasites be healthy and can someone become healthier or cured by purposefully colonizing oneself with worms?

The hygiene hypothesis suggested that modern life contributes to the proliferation of chronic disorders of the immune system, such as asthma, allergies, inflammatory bowel disease, and Crohn's. A broad range of supportive evidence has accumulated over the past two decades, showing that children who are exposed to farms are less likely to develop atopy or asthma, the rates of which have been increasing worldwide at great cost. In the past twenty years the hygiene theory has been refined and expanded to include the role of viruses, bacteria, gut flora, and parasites in training the immune system to distinguish between friend and foe. Mammals, parasites, and microbes coevolved for more than 100,000,000 years; until the twentieth century, infection of humans with parasites was nearly universal, with more than one billion people still infected worldwide (Weinstock and Elliott 2009). While certain parasitic infections can cause severe illness, anemia, or death (depending on which parts of the body they affect and how severe the infection is), the presence of parasites dampens inflammatory responses and may be necessary in developing and fine-tuning the immune response, especially in childhood. The exact mechanisms and pathways by which such infections modulate the human immune system are under scientific study. They involve Th- and T-cell responses and cytokines in ways not fully understood. Parasites release chemicals that allow them to evade the immune system by downregulating or dampening its sensitivity. In clinical trials for bowel disease, patients infected with helminths showed improvement. Recent evidence coming in about the healing potential for intestinal worms is encouraging, even exciting, for Crohn's, irritable bowel syndrome (IBS), multiple sclerosis, and severe autism, which is associated with gastrointestinal problems and repetitive behaviors that appear to stem, at least in part, from aberrant inflammatory responses. NIH-sponsored clinical trials for autism are underway at Mount Sinai School of Medicine (ClinicalTrials.gov 2009).

Worm therapy addresses the ill effects of the over-cleanliness problem at its source, restoring our disrupted ancestral unity with the biosphere and lower life forms by co-opting the worms' ability to inhibit inflammatory responses and immune hyper-responsiveness. Recent bioscientific studies at the University of Iowa and research centers worldwide indicate that intestinal fauna such as parasitic worms play a vital role in shaping the immune system's functional abilities. The positive outcomes of recent studies suggests that certain intestinal worms, specifically hookworms and whipworms, can be ingested medicinally to provide immunomodulatory benefits with minimal side effects. Not surprisingly, people suffering from chronic illnesses (Crohn's and IBD, allergies and autism) did not want to wait for final FDA approval, taking helminths therapeutically on their own, as alternative therapies, before conclusive results and risk reports were generated through the official pharmaceutical bureaucracy. Some scientists studying the effects of helminths in laboratory settings hope to isolate individual active substances that the parasites produce so that they may be marketed or synthesized to work on their own, and be made into standardized pharmaceutical products.

As a result of recent FDA rulings to limit public access to helminthic therapies and to grant TSO (*Trichuris suis ova* or pig whipworm eggs) investigational new drug status, Americans now travel to Mexico, Germany, or Thailand to get infected with worms under clinical supervision, or import them. TSO and hookworm (*Necator americanus*) are the preferred therapeutic worms because they do not spread beyond the gut and are unlikely to spread to other people. While very large numbers of worms could cause anemia, a moderate infection appears to have fatigue and abdominal discomforts as the main side effects. A therapeutic course that lasts ten weeks (using biweekly vials of 2,500 TSO eggs per dose or a one-time infection with hookworms through the skin) may cost from $3,000 to $5,000. Some sufferers apparently traveled to third-world countries to walk barefoot through raw sewage and acquire hookworms for free, reporting successful remission of their Crohn's symptoms on YouTube and Internet blogs. While some patients experienced rapid improvement upon infection, many have improved more gradually, for up to a year. The infections can last several years and can be easily eliminated with medication. The author of the blog "Worms to My Rescue!" Michelle Rowley (2010) describes the steady, gradual improvement of her numerous food allergies and intolerances since acquiring hookworms in April of the same year: "Hookworms are old medicine. I went into this treatment thinking that if I could just last three short months, I'd have my life back. That I'd eat a banana split and feel nothing at all. Modern medicine puts us into a mindset of quick, powerful results. Hookworm therapy is much more subtle, and requires patience I'm not used to."

Rowley (2010) explains that she has received many requests for "open-sourcing her infection" but she does not feel inclined to do so for the same reasons that, as a software developer, she does not agree with open-sourcing the software she designs or her OS X software or iTunes. It is very interesting and paradoxical that, while acknowledging that worms are "old medicine" she also speaks of the infection as similar to software, the flows of which follow legal guidelines and restrictions, as private intellectual property. While agreeing that open-sourcing of hookworms would be helpful to many, Rowley notes that she "licensed her infection" and this does not allow her to share. It is not clear whether the supplier of her infection had her sign a licensing agreement or whether she considers the infection to be her very own, thus her private property. The cost is definitely out of reach for poor Americans (and inhibitive for most). This recalls growing global equity issues emerging from the patenting and branding of seeds, plant varieties, and human genes, denounced by Vandana Shiva (2000) in her book *Stolen Harvest: The Hijacking of the Global Food Supply*. Shiva notes that free exchange of seeds and plants has been vital to traditional cultures ever since plant domestication was discovered, but new intellectual property laws criminalize free exchanges and cultivation/use of patented organisms and genes without compensation to the patent owner, often a powerful multinational corporation. The notion of licensing of intestinal worms reflects a grave and painful modern irony.

In her CNN column "Empowered Patient," Elizabeth Cohen's (2010) article "Man Finds Extreme Healing Eating Parasitic Worms" tells the story of a man who suffered with severe bowel disease that did not respond to medication and appeared likely to progress to bowel surgery. Because physicians did not agree to help him acquire the infection (it was not yet approved by the FDA), he traveled to Thailand to acquire pig whipworm eggs with the assistance of a Thai physician, who harvested them from a young girl. It was up to him to clean the eggs and grow them in a process called "embryonation." Upon his return to the United States he experienced complete remission of his severe bowel disease. He sought to have the infection and improvement documented by a medical researcher and the study was recently published in a scientific journal. The study and the publicity of it by the media are criticized by Dr. Stephen Hanauer (cited in Cohen 2010), chief of gastroenterology, hepatology, and nutrition at the University of Chicago, who stated that it is ridiculous and irresponsible to generalize based on one case and encourage people to pursue such treatments, as they may involve risks, particularly for immunosuppressed individuals, such as developing another type of infection. Other skeptics suggest that increased risk of cancer might occur with helminthic therapies over time, but there is yet no evidence in that regard (Cohen 2010).

The controversies surrounding worm therapy index manifold social, political, and economic ironies and cultural complexities, expressed in recent legal, medical, and ethical debates on medical authority and patient autonomy. Such struggles underlie the visible and invisible global circulation and global commodification of new biological therapies. An ancient symbiont of humans, the helminthic worm is being reclaimed as a miraculous solution to twenty-first-century plagues. Through legal, political, and medical processes a lowly parasite is now redefined as a drug, a situation that is drastically changing the flow of worms and wealth as well as the global flow of empowered persons seeking to render themselves more whole. This phenomenon is a very vivid illustration of how "alternative medicine" is constantly being constructed, reconstructed, negotiated, and embodied. Baer (2001:5) observed that "the relationship between biomedicine and alternative medical systems has been characterized by processes of annihilation, restriction, absorption and even collaboration." Having established its cultural supremacy in Western countries, biomedicine remains dominant by absorbing alternatives and reframing discussions in the language of risk.

The rise of alternative medicine is certainly tied to a resurgence in care for the self, a hallmark of other unorthodox healing movements of the past, such as the Popular Health Movement of the 1830s and 1840s in the United States, "a radical assault on medical elitism, and an affirmation of the traditional people's medicine." At the same time, there is already backlash from the political, commercial and biomedical establishment, manifested as efforts to control production and access to traditional and alternative medicines by adopting a public health rhetoric of "risk management." This is represented by the recent implementation of a European Union directive, passed in 2004, which demands that only traditional and herbal products that meet specific standards may be sold in stores. As a result, numerous popular herbal products have been taken off the shelves. According to Nigel Cassidy's (2011) BBC news report, many small producers say the directive is draconian and favors large manufacturers. Some anticipate losing their businesses, being unable to afford the fees. Authorities state that the rule is meant protect the public, although the new rules still do not require producers to prove that licensed products are effective, only that the standards were implemented.

Consumers and practitioners of alternatives periodically challenge the authority of biomedicine through market and Internet forces. The trend continues to be that alternatives struggle to gain legitimacy by aligning themselves with the standards of the dominant (hegemonic) system of biomedicine and professionalization of practitioners. But because of the hierarchical nature of capitalist societies and medical systems, these efforts reinforce the relatively weak status of alternative therapies and professionals. Nevertheless, there is a sea change that is taking place. Skeptics may view it primarily as absorption of holistic and traditional alternatives into the biomedical sphere for the purpose of controlling them, but the fact that there is more and more research being undertaken at the confluence of biomedicine and CAM (such as Harvard research on the neurobiology of touch and tai chi) will likely lead to a new type of medical practitioner in the future: someone who does not question the patient's right to look beyond the prescription pad or the operating room or scoff at the patient's need for healing in the absence of cure. Through the voices of patients who describe their healing journeys on the Internet, there is a grasp of the dynamic nature of pluralism and the personal and sensuous embodiment of suffering and healing experiences.

Subsequent chapters of this book invite the reader to further explore an array of traditions, methods, and experiences that share certain common features or emphases (dynamic flow in chapter 2, spirit and consciousness in chapter 3, and the senses in chapter 4), while at the same time highlighting the core problematic and argument of the book: the need for a reinvigoration of discourses and categories now used to label and analyze the experiences of health, illness, and healing as we move into the twenty-first century. Large-scale cultural trends and cross-cultural patterns are highlighted in each chapter, reflecting dominant themes suggested by the chapter titles, while diverse sources and case studies are used to shine an intimate light on the benefits and properties of traditional or alternative remedies and practices, many of which are becoming adapted or reconfigured as they are absorbed or enmeshed as "alternatives" into contemporary Western biomedical landscapes of possibilities and marketplaces of well-being.

Jeremy Carrette and Richard King (2005) critique popular Western discourses on "spirituality" as representing a silent takeover of "religion" and "Asian wisdom traditions" by the forces of the capitalist marketplace, which promote individualism and "consumerist spiritualities." Originally, Yoga and Taoism sought to extinguish self-centeredness and the attachment to material things, while fostering renunciation, compassion, and simplicity. Like self-help literature that discourages introspection or suffering, these traditions have been adapted and rebranded for Western tastes and agendas, becoming primarily tools for health, longevity, and professional achievement. Commercialization of yoga into a multimillion dollar industry, the growth of the yoga fashion and accessory industry, and the creation of yoga franchises such as Bikram Yoga aptly reflect this phenomenon. Biomedicine and modernity itself now stand to become transformed through this global flow of models and therapies. Old Eurocentric criteria and categories that have served science and capitalism faithfully for several centuries arguably need urgent revision. Carrette and King (2005:177) suggest that the wisdom and transformative potentialities of the world's traditional religious heritages may provide a vital resource to draw on in the effort to resist "unrestrained consumerism and the commodification of life itself." In the same spirit, I suggest that the dynamic global arena of interaction that we may loosely describe as "alternative medicine" can spur and support the creation of new forms of citizenship, embodiment, and consciousness. Hybrid therapies—various permutations of traditional medicine and biomedicine—may well engender opportunities for cultural transformations beyond the confines of Western bodies, markets, and popular imaginations, exposing the provisional quality of key categories and core principles of materialism and individualism, potentially leading to new epistemologies of health, healing, and caregiving.

Attempting an ambitious exploration of the confluence of traditional, Western and "alternative" medicine, this book will not concern itself with either proving or disproving the scientific validity of particular practices under discussion, or with fully summarizing characteristics or merits of specific treatments, methods, or techniques used for combating specific illnesses or promoting well-being. The emphasis is on the *social and cultural meaning and power* of "unorthodox" therapies and "traditional" healing principles, through particular studies or instances that demonstrate their instrumental and experiential salience to participants and communities. Close-ups and ethnographic case studies are juxtaposed with more general, historical, and cross-cultural insights and observations. The book calls the reader on a winding journey to examine diverse models and manifestations of health, illness, and healing in diverse contexts, where the local and the global cross paths, moving back and forth between the universal and the highly specific. While it may sometimes puzzle the reader seeking a sequential narrative or tidy classificatory scheme for sorting out CAM, this approach captures and expresses the distinctive strength (and also the messiness) of anthropology as a heuristic instrument: allowing time and space to shrink and dilate, collapse and expand, arrest and leap forward in the service of understanding human behaviors and social experiences in a complex, unique, and contingent way. At the intersection of the local and the global, the personal and the social, one is best able to note the distinctive and sometimes puzzling cultural underpinnings of healing, being drawn to expose and explore the fertile interconnections between mainstream and the margins from a global, holistic anthropological perspective.

QUESTIONS FOR CLASS DISCUSSION

1. Discuss your own experiences with the strengths and limitations of one or more unconventional therapies.
2. Discuss your own experiences with the strengths and limitations of biomedicine.
3. What are some possible incentives, advantages and disadvantages to biomedical physicians to offer alternative therapies to their patients within their own practice?
4. What are some possible incentives, advantages and disadvantages to providers of non-biomedical therapies to undergo licensing and professionalization?

QUESTIONS FOR ESSAY WRITING

1. Explore one of the Books of the Hippocratic Corpus at http://classics.mit.edu/ and reflect on remedies and recommendations. Which ones are still applicable today? Why?
2. Choose one of the leading natural therapies or health movements of the nineteenth century to research, summarize and reflect upon. How much of it has survived today?
3. Choose one of the following forces, elements or substances and research its health-related meanings, effects, and therapeutic uses in at least three different cultures: the sun, the moon, water, fire, earth, air, wind, rain, metal, wood, clay, gold, silver, wine, salt, oil.
4. Explore the history and traditional uses of a particular medicinal, hallucinogenic or food plant of your choice. Have uses changed over time? How is this plant viewed or used in your country? How has globalization changed local production and uses of it?

RECOMMENDED FILMS

Community Voices: Exploring Cross-Cultural Care through Cancer by Jennie Greene and Kim Newell, Harvard Center for Cancer Prevention: http://www.fanlight.com/catalog/films/329_cv.php.
Juliette of the Herbs by Tish Streeten: http://www.julietteoftheherbs.com/.
The Split Horn: Life of a Hmong Shaman in America by Taggart Siegel and Jim McSilver: http://www.pbs.org/splithorn/.

SUGGESTED READINGS

Baer, Hans A. (2004), *Toward an Integrative Medicine: Merging Alternative Therapies with Biomedicine*. Walnut Creek, CA: AltaMira Press.

Fadlon, Judith (2005), *Negotiating the Holistic Turn: The Domestication of Alternative Medicine*. Albany: State University of New York Press.

Lambert, Craig (2002), "The New Ancient Trend in Medicine," *Harvard Magazine* (March–April). http://harvardmagazine.com/2002/03/the-new-ancient-trend-in.html, accessed January 16, 2011.

INTERNET RESOURCES

Antiqua Medicina Exhibit at the University of Virginia: http://www.hsl.virginia.edu/historical/artifacts/antiqua/.

The Asclepion at Indiana University Bloomington: site devoted to Ancient Medicine: http://www.indiana.edu/~ancmed/intro.htm.

CAM Databases. The Research Council for Complementary Medicine (United Kingdom): http://www.rccm.org.uk/.

CAM on PubMed: http://nccam.nih.gov/research/camonpubmed/.

Creighton University Alternative Medicine: http://altmed.creighton.edu/default.htm.

Harvard Medical School Osher Research Center—Education: http://www.osher.hms.harvard.edu/education.asp.

Rosenthal Center for CAM at Columbia University: http://www.rosenthal.hs.columbia.edu/.

–2–

Substance, Energy, and Information Flows

Flow is a fundamental aspect of the natural world, the ultimate essence of life itself, a testimony to the dynamically complex nature of reality, and the basis of relationships. Everything that gives life and nourishes life must flow: rainwater, rivers, blood, semen, breast milk, nutrients, digestion, conversation, trade goods, and of course, the underlying quality of everything in the universe: that mysterious property of things called energy. The observable world depends upon the ebb and flow of winds, seasons, bodies of water, pollinating insects, and animal migrations to maintain and periodically restore itself. Like the circle of life metaphor or the notion of ecological balance, flow represents relation and interaction: the foundation of human beings' earliest and most intense relationships with one another and with the surrounding world. This is a classic concern of *cultural ecology*, a notion introduced by anthropologist Julian Steward in 1937, which has since expanded to encompass the full spectrum of interactions between societies and their environments, including local sustainability and global political economy (Porter 2001). The organizing theme of this chapter, *flow* is an empirically descriptive key term, a metaphorical tool for articulating life experiences and the quintessential vital principle.

In his landmark work on the Ndembu people of Zambia (central Africa), Victor Turner (1967:90) wrote: "If men and women are to beget and bear, suckle and dispose of physical waste they must enter into relationships—relationships which are suffused with the affective glow of the experiences." Such primordial experiences are fundamentally relational and alert us to relations in cosmos and society. The Ndembu speak of these processes as "rivers": the white, the red, and the black river. The three rivers and colors are multivocal ritual symbols that are linked to human physiology and cosmic realities: whiteness to milk and semen; red to blood and the many human experiences that involve the loss of it, particularly menstruation, birth, and aggression; and black to waste and decay. These are powers that underlie or constitute reality, connecting the divine with humans' inner nature and the natural world, the body being a microcosm of the universe and a template for mystical knowledge about the nature of things (Turner 1967:107).

Anthropologists have noted the centrality of flow, fluidity, and flux for the process of healing and for ensuring social well-being in African cultures (Masquelier 2001), Papua New Guinea (Strathern and Stewart 1999), and elsewhere, including the ancient medical traditions of India, China, and ancient Greece. Images of flow and circulation permeate the language of health and illness and reflect the basic human awareness that a flow of substances in the natural environment and the human body is needed for sustenance, survival, wellness, and healing. Harm ensues from lack of water, as well as too much water, an inadequate amount or variety of food, as well as excessive consumption of food, insufficient activity, but also overexertion, as well as temperature extremes. Indeed, these basic facts of life and health have been observed everywhere by humans, from the earliest times. Celebrated in the Latin poetry of Horace, the saying *aurea mediocritas* did not commemorate mediocrity as conceived today but the value of the golden mean between extremes. Going back to classical Greece, the middle road of moderation was considered a path of wisdom and longevity. Similar views found expression in Confucian and Buddhist philosophies of Asia. Modern scientific medicine widely acknowledges this as well, expressed in the notion of *homeostasis*: the state of internal balance attained by living things by regulation of physiological processes; sweating on a hot day lowers the body's temperature; in contrast, capillaries constrict when someone is cold in order to conserve heat and maintain internal temperature.

The awareness that natural ebbs and flows shape the environment and the human experience of health and sickness has existed in all cultures throughout the world from ancient times. All cultures have developed ways to capture and encode their knowledge and experience of how the living world functions and how humans should interact with their environment to maximize the well-being of local people in their community in order to preserve their ecological niche. Medical anthropologists and historians of medicine employ the term *humors* to refer to vital fluids, elements, or properties that cultures recognized as fundamental aspects of life. These must be kept in balance, often by means of consuming particular foods and liquids. While proper quantity is important (too much or too little of a vital fluid can cause illness), notions of hot/cold/cool and wet/dry play key roles in humoral balance, which may be assessed and interpreted differently in various healing traditions. Activities, weather changes, and emotions can deplete or restore these vital fluids, whereas traditionally prescribed foods, remedies, and behaviors can replenish them.

According to Andrew Strathern and Pamela J. Stewart (1999:35–41), the Melpa people of Papua New Guinea have an indigenous system based on two humors: blood and grease, which "form two separate but interconnected sources of vitality," and must flow freely and be exchanged appropriately for health and social harmony to be maintained and restored. Their properties and meaning in Melpa culture are complex and different in significant ways from European or biomedical notions of these substances. Both vital fluids can be depleted in people and communities: a man uses up his "grease" through intercourse and a woman through pregnancy and breast-feeding, for example, whereas blood can be "cooked" and dried up through intercourse, anger, sorcery, and other means, causing illness. To replenish grease in the body, one must consume pork fat and juicy vegetables, whereas eating certain local red fruit and red-stemmed greens restores blood. Strathern and Stewart observed that "the optimal conditions for health and fertility are found in the balancing of hot and cold in the cool" (1999:37). The fair-minded actions of a chief, described as "cool," are said to make grease for the group. Health and prosperity depend upon having these elemental life forces in the proper place, condition, and proportion, but it is equally vital to ensure their proper flow. Strathern and Stewart note that Melpa humors are analogs of wealth, which must flow between partners and kin to secure good relations. At the group level, exchanges of pigs are used to resolve conflicts (in payment for killings) and to promote and restore harmonious relations in the community.

Cross-culturally, beverages are commonly poured as offerings to ancestors and shared as key instruments of sociality and solidarity, helping support and enhance social connections and promote good health, as illustrated by the widespread practice of toasting someone's health. The flow of drinks, foods, gifts, and commodities and the essential and complex functions of circulation in establishing and strengthening social bonds and identities have been amply studied by anthropologists: from Malinowski's (1920) classic account of the *kula* ring, a ritualized exchange of prized shell armbands and necklaces in the Trobriand Islands (Papua New Guinea) to Mary Douglas and Baron Isherwood's (1996 [1979]) work on goods as an information system; from Sidney Mintz's (1985) landmark analysis of the social, economic, and political dimensions of the sugar trade to Daniel Miller's (1998) theory of shopping, and many other recent works on the flows of images, commodities, and humans—migrants, refugees, trafficked persons, and body parts—in the global marketplace (Ehrenreich and Hochschild 2002; Farr 2004; Ginsburg et al. 2002; Parreñas 2001; Scheper-Hughes and Wacquant 2002).

In writing about her fieldwork with Màwri society in Niger, Adeline Masquelier has deftly commented on the "vitality" of markets:

> Rather than being merely a "thing," in a reified sense, or a space of interaction and transaction, markets are animated with life and are personified. In the same manner that bodies are animated by the flow of substances within their boundaries, and in and out of their orifices, markets are endowed with life that is subject to the flux of people, the exchange of goods, and the circulation of news and values. (2001:209)

More importantly, she observed, the "health of a market" depends upon the presence of "spirits who protect it and animate it by their presence." Their involvement brings people in and gives power to the market: "[I]t is the sum of all these relations, material and spiritual, that gives *rai* (life) to the market" (Masquelier 2001:210). The prosperity of communities depends upon the flow of goods and persons, and the existence of sustaining relationships that connect the visible and the invisible worlds. Indeed, vital substances must be able to flow within living beings for good health and healing to occur, while goods and spirits must flow in and out of communities to ensure their health and prosperity.

Analogously, knowledge and information flow are necessary to ensure the survival and well-being of groups and social networks. It is widely known that the "vitality" and success of websites is measured by the number of "hits" they receive, reflecting the degree of Internet activity, commonly called "traffic." Similarly, active trading and regular fluctuations are key characteristics of healthy financial markets, the disruptions of which profoundly and dramatically impact nearly every institution and community in the contemporary world and the well-being of communities tied to the global economy. Such linkages between flux and vitality reflect the wide-ranging centrality of flows and exchanges in the natural and the social realms, from bodily and environmental movements to the movements of wealth, workers, viruses, or spirits, across visible or invisible boundaries, illustrating the symbolic overlap of distinct arenas of human experience.

In his exploration of local approaches to psychiatric practice in Argentine hospitals, Andrew Lakoff (2005:22) uses the terms *liquidity* and *circulatory networks* to describe the flow of bipolar patients' DNA from an Argentine psychiatric hospital to a French biotech company. The company had allied itself with several pharmaceutical companies and was building a DNA library in anticipation of discoveries linking a particular gene locus, representing a "patentable informational unit" (Lakoff 2005:160), with either disease vulnerability or medication response. By current international laws, such genomic discoveries constitute intellectual property and carry commercial rights. As Lakoff has eloquently observed:

> Popular discussions of globalization processes typically describe an increasingly rapid flow of information, capital, and human bodies across national borders in the wake of technological innovation and political-economic transformation. As a number of analysts have noted, however, such global circulation operate in relation to regulatory techniques and governmental strategies—at local, national, and transnational levels—that both encourage and constrain these flows. The negotiation of institutionalized regimes of coordination or harmonization—the linking of places through the creation of commensurable standards—is often necessary to make such circulation possible. (2005:41)

Another dark side of flows and circulation is aptly illustrated by articles such as Gillian Tett's (2009:6) "Icebergs and Ideologies: How Information Flows Fuelled the Financial Crisis," wherein she argues that the financial crisis of 2007 and 2008 was in part due to media and information flows that did not adequately reflect what was going on in the world of finance. An anthropologist who works as assistant editor for the *Financial Times*, Tett points to blind spots in media accounts of the financial world: mainstream media neglected certain aspects (the debt, credit, and derivatives market), which were perceived as boring (less conducive to "stories") as compared to the equity, currency, and commodity markets. This allowed bankers, politicians, and entrepreneurs to reap fat profits while a large part of the system was "submerged from sight, widely ignored" and protected from public scrutiny, like an iceberg (Tett

2009:6–7). The flow of information is intimately connected to the flow of resources, money, and power.

Access to knowledge and information is fundamental to survival: at the molecular and cellular level, life depends on the flow of chemical signals, such as electrolytes, enzymes, and hormones; being able to communicate the location of pollen-rich flowers is essential to the unity and survival of beehives—thus the intricate "dance" of the bees; communication about danger, mating, and food sources is essential to survival and reproduction for all living creatures, from microscopic insects to apes and blue whales. Anthropologically speaking, possession of valuable knowledge and information or access to these is associated with higher status in all societies. The key roles played in small-scale societies and mostly oral cultures by elders and ritual specialists (such as shaman-healers and story-tellers) in the transmission of valuable cultural and environmental knowledge have been increasingly supplanted by formally trained professionals, mass media, and the Internet in contemporary times. Thus, instead of learning from their mothers and grandmothers, women now turn to lactation consultants, books, and websites to gather information about breast-feeding and weaning their infants.

From the Flow of Rumors to Exposing the Global Traffic in Organs and Tissues

It is not only the flow of factual information that has real consequences, but the flow of rumors as well, as aptly illustrated in Abigail E. Adams's (1998) article "Gringas, Ghouls, and Guatemala," which examines the child-stealing scare of 1994, when rumors of organ theft from babies, accompanied by a $100 bill and a thank-you note in English, led to a series of violent attacks on foreigners, particularly U.S. women. Anxieties about strangers and the glaring inequalities of resources find expression in the flow of rumors, many of which contain elements of truth; the rumors may not be entirely factual, but certainly are embodiments of painfully felt social truths of inequality and impoverishment. In her 1996 article "Theft of Life: The Globalization of Organ-Stealing Rumors," Nancy Scheper-Hughes indicates that such rumors have been circulating since the 1980s in Brazil, Argentina, Colombia, Peru, Guatemala, Honduras, Mexico, and Korea. Since the 1990s such rumors have surfaced in Eastern Europe, Poland, Russia, Italy, and many parts of Africa, where they have been merged with stories of human vampires who steal blood for use in "magical medicine" or for sale to hospitals. Stray youngsters are said to be abducted and mutilated so that their organs feed the organ transplantation hunger of the "First World" with the bodies and lives of "Third World" babies and children. In her earlier work, Scheper-Hughes suggested that the stories were true at "that indeterminate level between fact and metaphor," manifesting the violence of daily life in the poorest neighborhoods, the grotesque interplay of medical, economic, and social relations being felt "at the immediate level of the violated and dismembered body" (Scheper-Hughes 1996:5).

The reality described by Scheper-Hughes (1996:6) speaks of two Brazils: one of the very poor, whose bodies are often injured by Third World medical maltreatment (teeth pulled that could be filled, faces scarred by and limbs amputated for treatable conditions, unnecessary deaths due to hospital-acquired infections, dead bodies claimed by the state for dissection), and that of the middle and upper classes, who avail themselves of the latest medical therapies and technologies: body sculpting, plastic surgery, and transplants, including use of "eye banks" reserved for the wealthy. Returning to this book's theme of "alternative medicine," it is necessary to recognize that in a context such as this, the medical world of the poor and the biomedical world of the wealthy are two alternative and parallel medical realities. Such a dual biomedical reality is common throughout the "developing world," where high-quality and high-tech biomedicine is an unaffordable and tightly guarded resource accessible only to a segment of the population. The world in which poor people live is not simply one of traditional healing practices and magical beliefs but one of alternative opportunity and risk, biomedically speaking, which they are unable to control. Whether or not poor kids are kidnapped for their organs to be recycled, Scheper-Hughes writes:

> The organ stealing rumor has its basis in poor people's perceptions, grounded in a social and biomedical reality, that their bodies and those of their children might be worth more dead than alive to the rich and powerful. They can all too easily imagine that their bodies, and the bodies of their young children, may be eyed longingly by those with money. As poor people in shantytowns see it, the ring of organ exchange proceeds from the bodies of the young, the poor, and the beautiful to the bodies of the old, the rich and the ugly, and from poor nations in the South to rich nations in the North. (1996:7)

The author notes that the timing of child kidnapping and dismemberment rumors arose and spread in South America and South Africa during politically violent times, when military regimes committed acts of extreme violence against local people and abuses were performed by authorities against civilians, including medical professionals, such as kidnappings, mutilations, and "disappearances," which contributed to a justified sense of alarm and "bodily, ontological insecurity." One of the few weapons of the weak in cases of extreme social suffering, these rumors accurately reflect a global reality in which the poor are devalued and dispossessed, their life-force captured to feed the needs of the rich and powerful. In the absence of human rights safeguards, legal protections for organ donors, and a fair health care system, people have legitimate reasons to be suspicious of authorities and the promises of high-tech medicine. In the absence of social trust, transplantation technology is another potential tool for oppression.

The human body and its parts have been transformed into commodities through modern medicine and globalization, from corneas to tendons, from women's eggs to stem cells, from blood to DNA; tissues can nowadays be "rendered liquid," in financial terminology, to be banked and sold to the highest bidder, often thousands of miles away. According to writer and anthropologist Scott Carney (2010b), one in four Hindu pilgrims to the Tirumala temple in Andhra Pradesh donate their hair to Venkateswara, the god of the temple, which is then sold for millions of dollars annually. The temple is the world's top supplier of the pricey "remy hair," now used in the most exclusive salons in America to create hair extensions, weaves, and wigs for celebrities, and is responsible for almost a third of the Indian trade. Until the 1960s the temple used to burn the hair it collected, but auctions have since become "cutthroat affairs" among resellers, where millions of dollars change hands. Since then, the price of the best quality hair has gone up tenfold, hovering below US$200 per kilogram in 2010. Hair is obtained from the floors of barber shops, and long-haired women's combs are often acquired and resold by peddlers, who eke out a living this way. The discarded hair ends are used in the production of fertilizer and L-cysteine, an amino acid used to supplement baked goods. Such activities amount to a shocking figure of 900 billion dollars in the global hair trade, in which India plays a key role (Carney 2010b).

The term *donation* and the rhetoric of gift-giving widely used in reference to blood and other tissues tends to obscure the fact that many of the givers are poor and undercompensated. Research subjects or "human guinea pigs" can earn extra income, and some make a living by volunteering as research study participants in the testing of new drugs and procedures. Advocates have argued that the minimal payments inadequately compensate for the long-term risks and health consequences of being a human research subject. At the same time, some subjects earn more than US$50,000 annually. Guinea-pigging is becoming a twenty-first-century "alternative lifestyle," a source of global community, inspiration for memoir-writing and social critique, and a postmodern career path, as illustrated by the presence of the online magazine *Guinea Pig Zero: A Journal for Human Research Subjects* (guineapigzero. com), which describes itself as an "occupational jobzine for people who are used as pharmaceutical or medical research subjects." The buying and selling of organs for transplantation is illegal in most countries at this time (although some authorities have suggested that "fair payment" may alleviate the shortage of organs), whereas the buying of plasma, blood, sperm, and other tissues for research tends to be remunerated modestly.

Not surprisingly, certain populations and minorities who need cash and have fewer opportunities for employment tend to form the majority of donors. Whereas blood bank donations are typically unpaid, plasma donations are paid, and there appear to be no ill effects from donating plasma, at least not in the short term. According to Andrew Pollack (2009), many Mexican plasma donors fly across the border from Mexico into the United States to donate; thus a number of plasma collection facilities are located along the U.S.–Mexico border. A woman donating twice a week may earn as much as her working husband ($60/week). The plasma is then used to produce drugs like IVIG (intravenous immune globulin), used to treat immune deficiencies, albumin for burn and trauma victims, and clotting protein therapies for hemophilia that may cost US$100,000–$350,000 annually (Pollack 2009). Multiple lawsuits have been filed against plasma product companies, including a class-action suit by several hospitals. Plasma companies have become few and very powerful internationally (five companies in 2009), driving plasma prices up as demand increased. The Federal Trade Commission filed a lawsuit that blocked a planned acquisition by the plasma-drug industry, describing the industry as a "tight oligopoly with a high level of information sharing" (Pollack 2009). There is a global shortage of all human tissues for transplantation and for medical research. Some governments have suggested making all citizens into donors, unless they fill out a form to opt out. Many poor people are fearful that their death may be hastened or provoked to obtain coveted organs and tissues. Since the buying and selling of these is a recent phenomenon, legislation is absent or unclear in many countries, leaving an open arena for underground marketing and exploitation of both donors and recipients. Desperate, impoverished people who struggle to support their families may see themselves as collections of spare parts that can be exchanged for cash in the global market. It is important to reflect on the directions of tissue and cash flows and where the profit and capital accumulates in this global flow of vital fluids and funds.

Poor women in India and other developing countries can offer their bodies as surrogate mothers in exchange for cash to support their families (Carney 2010a). At the same time, young Western university women may sell their eggs on the Internet for amounts many times what Third World surrogates get for a ten-month lease of their bodies. Like the value of "spare" children who are offered for international adoption and the value of children produced through modern technologies of conception (such as IVF and surrogate motherhood), these new flows of vital tissues and financial resources are embedded in global politics of inequality as well as local realities that are outcomes of modern capitalist and biomedical development that draw upon the "resources" of peripheral nations and less powerful people(s) as labor and capital. As their lands and waters have been claimed, developed, and polluted by governments and businesses, indigenous people have become increasingly limited in their ability to produce what they need for their own survival and increasingly drawn to (and needful of) money to access basic resources. As native people seek to enter the global flows of cash and power by any means that they can, the commodification of body parts is but one aspect of the new transnational networks through which life forces and resources flow. They represent a new form of global cannibalism or vampirism rooted in socioeconomic and political realities. Thus, from the perspective of critical anthropology and sociology, one must question the "gift of life" narrative in light of the "theft of life" rumors and recognize that the existence of "spare" organs, the "scarcity" of transplant organs and the "shortage" of organs are recent social constructions: the creations of late twentieth-century global consumerism, biotechnological progress, and socioeconomic inequalities. These practices are also manifestations of a cultural trend of denial of death, expressed in the willingness to pay large sums and take surgical risks to stay young and live beyond the limits of the flesh.

Nancy Scheper-Hughes (1996:9) denounced this "scarcity" of organs as "a new form of medical *iatrogenesis*: a harmful effect of modern medical care that is based, in this case, upon a 'rapacious need,'" borrowing Margaret Lock's evocative words. Organ theft accounts were long dismissed as "urban legends" by authorities, particularly in the United States, where buying and selling organs remains illegal. However, after almost two decades of investigative anthropological activism on these issues, Nancy Scheper-Hughes's research in organ trafficking has contributed to international recognition of the exploitative nature of organ harvesting and the transnational flow of organs from poor to the wealthy. Her efforts led to the creation of the international task force Organ Watch and the successful arrest of a number of organ dealers, thus putting a roadblock in the contemporary traffic flow of body parts. These dealers have been operating within a global network that "harvests" Third World organs for wealthy Western consumers. Poor donors are commonly cheated or paid reduced amounts for their body parts, which are then sold for high profits; medical follow-up care is frequently unavailable; and legal safeguards or recourse are not available or accessible to the poor. Her detective work assisted in securing U.S. cooperation that culminated in the 2009 arrest of a key organ broker in New York City, Levy-Izhak Rosenbaum, who had been involved for many years in a global organ procurement ring.

Duality of Water: Vitality and Contamination

Not surprisingly, the 2010 meetings of the American Anthropological Association, taking place in legendary New Orleans, at the mouth of the Mississippi River, were devoted to the notion of "Circulation" as the annual theme, a tribute to the expanding relevance and power of the metaphor of circulation for exploring the intricate ties of the local and the global in the contemporary world. C. J. Thompson (1929:4) observed that people seem "to have regarded water as a thing of mystery," as both "divine essence" and "supreme cleanser," endowed with supernatural powers and healing properties. Bodies of water like the Nile, Euphrates, Ganges, and Jordan rivers were considered sacred. Thus, in the Christian tradition, purification and baptism by water exemplifies the connection of cleanliness and holiness, which had been long established throughout the ancient world. In Ireland, Holy Well visitation is a regular part of parish life and may cure a variety of ills, including headaches, abdominal pain, warts, whooping cough, sore throats, or eye problems, for which people may keep a small bottle in the pantry (Ray 2010).

Water has been used for healing as well as ritual purification (ablution) in many cultures. The use of saliva as medicine appears in the Bible, the Talmud, and among the Romans and early Arab physicians for a variety of purposes, but chiefly as an antidote to the bites of snakes and dogs (Thompson 1929:212). Hippocrates recommended baths for healing. From ancient Rome to Turkey to Japan, public baths and mineral waters constituted an important part of the culture and social life. Rainmaking rituals were found in Ancient Egypt and among Native Americans like the Zuni, but also in rural Romania (*Paparuda*). Water is beautiful and life-giving. It is a great force of nature, often unpredictable and uncontrollable. The danger of excessive rain damaging crops, the danger of flooding, the danger of storms, particularly for fishermen, and the danger of drowning are nowadays compounded by the post-pasteurian knowledge that water is a common source of contamination with bacteria, parasites, and environmental toxins, and the modern fact of inadequate access to clean and safe water for millions of people living in poverty.

A central Apache myth of creation describes their culture hero, White Painted Woman, emerging gradually from the water. In religions worldwide, women are often associated with water and the cycles of the moon that are connected to the movement of tides and the cycles of fertility. Not coincidentally, the word month comes from the word moon. In many cultures, female water spirits are a source of danger, particularly for men, such as the mermaids of Ancient Greece. Represented by a serpent, the female deity known as Mami Wata is propitiated throughout Africa and the African diaspora. She is beautiful, seductive, protective, and life-threatening, but also a bringer of good fortune and associated with money and capitalist prosperity (Drewal 2008). Water is of course present in many humoral systems (Greek and Islamic Humoralism, Ayurveda, as well as Traditional Chinese Medicine), commonly as an element in a wet/dry dyad that needs to be remain balanced, since both overabundance and depletion are dangerous states.

Water is associated with the yin principle in Chinese yin/yang cosmology, which dates back at least two thousand years and describes the universe as being in a state of dynamic equilibrium between two complementary natural forces: *yin* (contractive, centripetal, responsive, positive, cold, and wet) and *yang* (expansive, centrifugal, demanding, negative, hot, and dry). For this equilibrium and health to be maintained, the life principle *chi* or *qi* must be allowed to flow unimpeded or restored through various therapeutic methods, especially foods and herbs but also acupuncture, the insertion of fine needles along the body's energy channels known in English as the "meridians," and purposeful restorative movement such as tai chi and qigong. Spaces and interiors can also become unbalanced, a matter addressed in the practice of feng shui, which uses particular colors and objects along with criteria related to the four directions and their symbolic significance to restyle and reorganize living and working spaces for greater harmony and prosperity. According to this view of the universe, the human person is an integral part of nature and subject to the same natural laws. In the graphic representation of yin/yang, each contains the seed of the other. Things are integrated and interdependent in such a way that no part can function in abstraction of other parts or ignorance of the whole (Scheper-Hughes and Lock 1987).

In his influential account of the history of madness in Europe, Michel Foucault (1988 [1965]:166–72) vividly described the polyvalent uses of water immersion and showers as remedies for severe mental illnesses in eighteenth- and nineteenth-century France, alternately cooling, heating, moistening, or drying the humors as it strengthened the temperament. The cold water cure or hydropathy became popular in nineteenth-century Britain, being most popular among the upper classes, especially for "diseased savants, sick poets and poorly novelists" like Tennyson or Darwin (Bradley 2002:25). Some hydropathic practitioners were medically educated and some were not. Many members of the orthodox medical profession attacked hydropathy, offended in part by the fact that its discoverer, Vincent Priessnitz, was a Silesian "peasant," yet the orthodox opposition was not unanimously against hydropathy. The cure was believed to work by stimulating the body to heal itself. Some perceived it as a spiritual phenomenon.

Current Practice: Homeopathy *and Ayurveda*

Water played an important role in many of the "unorthodox" practices that were flourishing in nineteenth-century Europe, including mesmerism and homeopathy. Homeopathy has grown tremendously since its birth 250 years ago and has gained international scope, with particular popularity in India, where it exhibits some affinities with Ayurveda.

In the words of Frank and Ecks (2004), Indian homeopathy has been indigenized as a non-colonial form of modern medicine, becoming creatively tailored to local contexts and needs, with more than 100,000 college-trained homeopaths practicing throughout India and almost twice as many overall. Homeopathy is part of a rich array of complementary therapies in many urban areas such as Oaxaca, Mexico, its non-invasive approach appealing particularly to women, who tend to monitor their health and that of their families (Whiteford 1999). In Mexico, as in India and the European Union, most practitioners hold conventional medical school degrees, followed by subsequent specialization.

Homeopathy continues to be popular worldwide, despite having had a significant downturn in the face of the competition over the past 100 years and facing sustained animosity from allopathic medicine practitioners. In 2005 and 2007, the leading UK journal *The Lancet* published articles stating that homeopathy worked no better than placebo and made false claims, and that the National Health Service would be cutting back on funding to leading homeopathic providers. The term *allopathic medicine* (commonly used for conventional biomedicine) was originally coined to distinguish it from homeopathic medicine, emphasizing a therapeutic approach that relies primarily on treatment by opposites rather than treatment by similars. The Greek root word *allos* means different; *homoios* means similar; *pathos* refers to suffering or passion.

Homeopathy was founded by German physician Samuel Hahnemann (1755–1843) and provided a gentle alternative to the heroic medical practices of the day. The *materia medica* of homeopathy comprises thousands of substances from plant, animal, mineral sources, or even the disease itself, which are diluted until virtually undetectable. In choosing remedies that mirror the symptoms experienced by the sufferer, homeopathy seeks to aid the healing process rather than suppress the symptoms. Thus, the popular remedy *Apis mellifica* is made from bee venom and commonly used for bee stings as well as other bright red manifestations accompanied by swelling, burning, and sharp stinging sensations, including rashes and tonsillitis. The less of the original substance that remains, the higher the potency; therefore a 3 C dilution is more limited in action than 30 C, which acts less deeply than 100 C. The more a remedy has been diluted the longer and deeper it acts, and fewer doses are required (Ullman 1991 [1988]:12). The use of dilutions above 30 C (in the hundreds or thousands) is the province of trained homeopathic practitioners.

Homeopathy's key principles are the *principle of similars* (like cures like) and the *principle of infinitesimals* (greater dilutions have deeper effects). It relies upon two techniques of preparation: *potentization* (multiple dilutions) and *succussion* (firm striking of the vial against a leather pad or the palm of one's hand). Water is used to dilute the active ingredient multiple times until only the energetic signature or "memory" of the original substance remains in the fluid; for the solid preparations, the key substance is ground with lactose. The remedy can be consumed in liquid form or prepared as small lactose-based tablets, pellets, or granules. When administered, one to five of these are held under the tongue. As exemplified in the work of Dana Ullman (1991 [1988]), classical homeopathy is an approach that administers only one carefully selected "constitutional" remedy at a time fit to a client's "bodymind" type. The "right remedy" is determined in an elaborate interview, which alternately resembles clinical case-taking and psychotherapy, and it is based upon the totality of a person's symptoms: physical, mental, emotional, and social. An interesting new homeopathic case-taking tradition has emerged based upon the work of Indian homeopath Rajan Sankaran, "the sensation method," which guides the patients' verbal descriptions and expressions of discomfort to elicit sensation words (like tight, sharp, or burning) that are then used to identify a unique remedy for each patient (Hpathy.com 2011).

At the heart of homeopathy is the notion of vital force, energetic and informational in nature, which may be restored or enhanced by careful prescribing of a constitutional remedy that fits the patient's experience precisely. This comprehensive approach is based upon an understanding that water, plants, animals, minerals, chemical substances, textures, colors, sounds, behaviors, thoughts, emotions, and life circumstances (past and present) are complexly and intimately interconnected through webs of homeopathic relationships. Remedies are divided into three kingdoms, the Minerals (including the Periodic Table of Elements), the Plants, and the Animals, and further into subclasses based on characteristics (metals, fungi, spiders, and so on), each member having its own distinguishing personality traits and constitutional issues. Homeopaths can make their own remedy out of any substance. Colors and musical sound remedies have been used homeopathically to rebalance organs and *chakras*. The restoration of life force at the microscopic level is intimately tied to equilibrium at the cosmic level, constituting the basis for personal health and vital balance in homeopathy.

Energy, Life-Force, and the Powers of the Sun

Constantly changing energy is the basic process that underlies life, human, animal, and vegetal. As noted by Nobel Prize–winning physicist Richard Feynman, the concept of energy is not itself explanatory. Its ultimate nature eludes us. To say that a wind-up toy moves because of energy is not inherently scientific; instead, saying that someone's hand wound up the spring inside, which then made it move by uncoiling itself is a scientific explanation. The transformations and effects of energy have been well documented scientifically, as has the fact that, at the smallest level, energy comes in discrete bundles. Although we may not think about this on a daily basis, most energy circulating on earth, from the movement of air and water to the nutrient and glucose content of plant foods, or the concentrated power in fossil fuels, derives from the heat and light of the sun, the provider of abundant (yet not necessarily inexhaustible) energy, which is captured, stored, transformed, and ultimately dissipated by both animate and inanimate things in myriad ways. Not surprisingly, the sun was considered a god in many cultures and mythologies, such as the Aztec Empire, where it was believed that the flow of blood from human sacrifices was required to keep the sun moving. King Louis XIV of France was referred to as "the sun king." Like many royalty, he claimed divine right to power and aspired to embody the utmost grandeur in his displays of authority. Currently, the term *sun worshipper* is ironically applied to persons who love sunbathing, as controversies about risks versus benefits of sun exposure create divisions between sun-shunning dermatologists and sun advocates, who tout its profound healing powers.

Traditional notions of the sun as divine giver of life and the sun as healer have been counteracted in recent decades by widespread fear of the harmful effects of the sun's ultraviolet rays. Most Westerners are keenly aware of the link between sunburn and skin cancer (as well as wrinkles and age spots) and have been strongly persuaded, if not indoctrinated, that most sun exposure must be avoided at all costs. Dire warnings and elaborate guidelines for sun avoidance have been issued by the biomedical establishment, led in the United States by the American Academy of Dermatology, in collaboration with popular media and the cosmetics industry. However, there is growing evidence that the avoidance of the sun by modern urban dwellers may have negative health consequences. A well-established connection exists between vitamin D and bone development, as well as bone pain and bone loss. Low levels of vitamin D, reaching epidemic proportions in the northern hemisphere, are being evaluated by scientists as a potential contributor to modern ills such as multiple sclerosis, autism, and internal cancers that have been increasing at northern latitudes (Khalsa 2009; Hobday 1999).

As Westerners retreat indoors, covering themselves head-to-toe with sunscreens, they may be going against a biologically evolved need for sunlight. Anthropologically speaking, humans spent most of their evolutionary history in Africa, hunting and gathering on foot, with minimal clothing, a stark contrast to the modern lifestyle. The hormone vitamin D is produced by the skin in ample amounts in response to regular sun exposure. People who avoid the sun and darker-skinned people (who make less of it) may easily develop an insufficiency, especially if living in cloudy areas, away from the equator. Dietary sources alone do not appear to be adequate, but recommendations for vitamin D are currently being revised upward for children and adults, since they appear to have been set much too low originally. Thus, the "sunlight vitamin" has made a dramatic entrance into the contested field of preventive medicine. Since the debut of the new millennium, family practitioners and endocrinologists have begun to test their patients' vitamin D levels, prescribing mega-dose supplements to correct deficiencies. At the same time, unorthodox medicine advocates have been issuing warnings about yet unknown long-term dangers of using chemical sunscreens in excess, and calling for a return to the sun, in moderation.

Encountered under a multitude of name labels and local definitions, the concept of life force or vital energy plays a central role in the field of alternative medicines, both Eastern and Western, either explicitly (the *qi* of Traditional Chinese Medicine or the "vital force" of homeopathy) or implicitly, as the influence of massage, rhythm, movement, sound, or color (explored in chapter 4). Common manifestations of energy are heat, light, kinetic (motion), mechanical, electrical, thermal, atomic, nuclear, and potential energy. The science of physics states that energy behaves according to precise laws and principles. It further states that energy can be transformed from one type into another type but cannot be either created or destroyed; the total amount of energy remains unchanged. This is known as the first law of thermodynamics. Another interesting property of energy is its equivalency or interchangeability with mass: Einstein's famous equation $E = mc^2$ showed energy and mass to be equivalent forms, where mass is the amount of matter contained in an object. Embodiments of energy, various substances are particular kinds of matter, each one having uniform properties and a definite composition by weight. Water, salt, human blood, or homogenized honey are examples of substances, although in common speech the term *substance* is used to index a much broader range of things, from DNA to material wealth, to the content or kernel of a conversation. Whereas the continuity and unity between matter and energy has only been recognized and formulated in Western science in the twentieth century, it is both a cosmic and an experiential reality long acknowledged cross-culturally, finding expression and application in a variety of cultures and indigenous healing traditions, such as the heat-generating healing dances of !Kung San people of sub-Saharan Africa, which may date back 30,000–100,000 years B.C.E., to the bodily energy centers referred to as *chakras* in India's Ayurvedic medical tradition, possibly originating as far back as 4000 B.C.E.

Energy manifests itself in many forms and changes from one form to another, tending toward dispersion or entropy. At the smallest level, molecules, atoms, and subatomic particles bounce and vibrate: in a hot cup of liquid, molecules move very fast and collide with one another and the walls of the container, releasing their energy as heat. Heat release indicates a flow of energy as the liquid cools. Energy tends to flow from a high concentration or intensity to a lower one, but it can be blocked, pushed back, stored, or released suddenly. We know energy by its effects. In the arena of energy-based alternative healing, energy loss manifests as illness and practitioners use various methods to rebalance, store, or replenish the energy of a person, the energy of particular organs, or unblock energy flow using particular points and channels of the patient's body, which vary (yet overlap significantly) across different traditions, from the Maya to the Chinese.

Changes and flows of energy that make *everything* happen, notes David Watson (2005), author of an insightful and entertaining website for science and technology education. This "Mysterious Everything," as he calls it, "flows in bite-sized chunks (literally) through life, from one living thing to another living thing to another living thing, and so on and so on," eventually spreading out as unusable heat. While its ultimate origin remains elusive for scientists and a point of contemplation for theologians and mystics, the interpretations and applications of energy in both conventional and unconventional medicine have been enormously diverse: the use of electrocardiograms and electroencephalograms, which gather valuable electrical information about the functioning of the heart and the brain, nutritional supplements and diets aimed at modulating metabolism, acupuncture needles placed along particular energy channels to relieve pain and anxiety, Native American sweat lodge ceremonies to transform consciousness and induce healing experiences, or the hot/cold or wet/dry properties of foods, spices, and techniques, which are conceptualized differently in many societies, but widely recognized for their ability to address health imbalances.

Energy medicine is one of the types of alternative medicine recognized by the NCCAM (2011). This places it in a separate category from the use of foods, herbs, and nutrition, which it identifies as biologically based. Even though modern physics has demonstrated the equivalence of matter and energy at the subatomic level, the healing practices that tend to be grouped together under the title of "energy medicine" continue to be regarded with greater suspicion by biomedical practitioners, as being more esoteric and more difficult to explain, measure, and substantiate, and lagging behind the other healing modalities in achieving recognition and legitimacy. An exception has been the energy-based practice called *reiki*, a recent offshoot of this approach that is becoming widely known as "therapeutic touch" or "healing touch," and making important inroads into biomedical settings throughout the developed world. I studied the Radiance Technique method of reiki during my anthropological fieldwork in Romania in 1998, an experience I explore in more detail in chapter 4.

Nourishment and Healing

Three to four millennia B.C.E., the ancient Sumerians, Egyptians, and Babylonians had ample knowledge of plants, medicines, and embalmment, bestowed by the gods, who were thought of as great healers. Discharges from their bodies transformed into healing plants and oils, such as olive and cedar. In his book on the history of the apothecary, C. J. Thompson (1929:13) described the existence of Egyptian papyri dating back to 1850 B.C.E. with medical prescriptions "the ingredients of which consist mostly of herbs, dates, onions, beer, milk, oil and honey." However, the Papyrus Ebers (dating to 1500 B.C.E.) detailed a *material medica* of 700 different substances, animal, mineral, and vegetal, such as aloes, coriander, myrrh, opium, celery, pomegranate, and peppermint, which could be taken internally as "decoctions, infusions, pills, confections, boluses, draughts, cakes, lozenges, powders and inhalations" (Thompson 1929:13). Plant medicines were used to induce vomiting and urination, and some were administered as enemas, poultices, and ointments.

In adapting to a wide range of environments, humans have developed a variety of subsistence strategies for satisfying their needs. A biocultural approach to the relationship between food and health acknowledges that human biology, the natural environment, and culture play equally significant roles in shaping human behavior with regard to food, whether used as nourishment, medicine, or both. Anthropological studies have shown that people in small-scale subsistence economies use a broad range of resources in their environments, consuming diets that are nutritionally rich and provide adequate nutrient content (vitamins, minerals, carbohydrates, proteins, and fats) and calories for their needs. Based upon hunting, fishing, and gathering, the earliest known form of human livelihood, foraging diets typically include a wide range of plant and animal foods (including some insects) and appear to have been nutritionally sufficient as long as the range of movement and foraging activities of the group were not impeded, as they have been in modern times through colonialism, development, and globalization. In her popular article, "The Inuit Paradox," Patricia Gadsby (2004) reflects on the puzzling fact that Inuit Eskimo of the Arctic Circle living on traditional high-fat, high-protein foods have much better cardiovascular health than the average North American today. The food sources the Inuit relied upon before their diets became increasingly Westernized included delights such as raw fish, seal oil, and whale skin, and as a special treat, a mix of berries and whipped fat resembling ice cream. When they engaged in the arduous labor of subsistence hunting and gathering, people living in the far north were not faced with a need to lose weight, like sedentary modern people consuming energy-dense, high-carbohydrate, industrially processed foods but were instead faced with the challenge of keeping weight on during the long and frigid winters in order to avoid seasonal late-winter starvation, when the meat of wild animals became too lean.

The Inuits' locally adapted way of life was characterized by a conspicuous scarcity of vegetable foods and sunlight and by a primary reliance on meat, fat and skin of marine mammals, berries, and seaweed. But despite its apparent imbalance of "major" food groups (a concept that for decades has remained at the heart of U.S. public health campaigns in nutrition and its food pyramid models), the traditional Inuit diet provides sufficient vitamins (including A, C, and D) and minerals, along with a much lower risk of vascular and chronic disease than modern diets. A key ingredient accounting for the circulatory benefits of the Inuit diet has been identified: monounsaturated omega-3 fatty acids, such as those found in fish oil and flax oil. These unsaturated fats and the fats of wild animals are qualitatively different from saturated fats that predominate in the bodies of domesticated land mammals and dairy products, fats that have been shown to clog arteries and promote inflammation, or the "trans fats" produced industrially by hydrogenating vegetable oils to make them more solid and extend product shelf life, which have been shown to significantly contribute to vascular blockage. Increasingly popular as dietary supplements and recommended nowadays by Western medical practitioners and researchers, omega-3 fats have a beneficial effect on blood cholesterol and triglycerides, reduce the viscosity of blood, and tame inflammatory processes that contribute to common chronic ailments of industrialized societies such as heart disease, arthritis, and diabetes (Gadsby 2004). This Inuit paradox describes what I call the *alternative medicine paradox:* much of what is promoted and consumed as cutting-edge alternative medicine remedies and therapies is elsewhere time-tested cultural knowledge. Northern European grandmothers have been giving their grandchildren cod liver oil in the winter for centuries, but it is only recently that such popular practices are becoming vetted in the public arenas of laboratories and markets.

Throughout most of our evolutionary history, people have lived on diets that included a diversity of plant sources greater than what characterizes people who depend on agricultural production and market economies, who tend to consume diets that are energy-dense, high in complex carbohydrates and processed fats, and include only a handful of plant and animal species on a regular basis. According to Richard Lee's study of the Dobe Ju/'hoansi (!Kung San) people of the northwest Kalahari in the late 1960s and early 1970s, the !Kung had "an astonishing inventory of 105 edible plants: 14 fruits and nuts, 15 berries, 18 species of edible gum, 41 edible roots and bulbs, and 17 leafy greens, beans, melons and other foods," and were successfully able "to feed themselves by an average of about 20 hours of subsistence work per adult per week" (2003:40). Hunted meat and mongongo nuts each contributed approximately 30 percent of the diet, ensuring an adequate amount of protein. Missing in the !Kung diet thirty years ago were refined carbohydrates. Not surprisingly, heart disease was rare as well. In contrast, by the 1990s, the Ju/ people had become settled in villages and dependent upon cultivated grains and food relief, alcohol, cigarettes, and "vast quantities of heavily-sugared tea whitened with powdered milk"; their health declined significantly (Lee 2003:170). As they adapt to the world system, indigenous people struggle to maintain their cultural identity. New forms of grassroots social action and strategies of subsistence emerge as they reclaim ancestral lands and struggle to rejuvenate their culture and communities.

Nutritional variety decreased, while chronic and epidemic illnesses became increasingly common as food production and animal domestication became widespread 10,000 years ago. Food producers claimed the more fertile areas of land and foragers were relegated to marginal environments, where they survived until recently. Pastoralists rely upon domesticated animals for a significant portion of their nutritional needs, using milk and milk products (particularly fermented ones) as their main source of nutrition, and only occasionally sacrificing animals for meat. Some contemporary pastoralists cultivate or purchase grains. Increasingly common is the change from "high-milk and mixed-species pastoralism" to sedentary life and a diet of high fat and high carbohydrates, which has a negative impact on health (Etkin 2006:19).

Industrialization brings on an initial improvement in the flow of resources and waste, documented cross-culturally, as year-round access to food supplies and sanitation improve, contributing to decreases in child mortality and greater life expectancies, followed by reduced birth rates. This demographic transition is followed by a change in morbidity and mortality patterns (causes of sickness and death, respectively) from infectious disease to "diseases of civilization" such as cancer, arthritis, diabetes, asthma, allergies, and various other disorders of the immune system. While individuals still succumb to infections, at the population level the patterns change with development to a "modern disease profile," a process known as the health transition or the epidemiological transition (Weitz 2010:24). On the bleaker side, with the advent of market capitalism, social and health inequalities have continued to increase worldwide along with the dependence of indigenous people on wage labor and energy-dense consumer products: processed foodstuffs, alcoholic beverages, cigarettes, ready-made apparel, pharmaceuticals, and mass media (Weitz 2010; Singer and Baer 2007).

Global food politics and food insecurity present urgent concerns (FAO 2000). Nearly 800 million people worldwide face food deficits, the majority of whom are poor, and more than 100 million children under five are underweight; stunting among young children has been decreasing globally since 1990, particularly in Asia, but it appears to be increasing in Africa; globally, one in three people is malnourished and billions lack regular access to safe water and sanitation (WHO 2001a,b, 2010). Half of childhood deaths can be attributed either directly or indirectly to malnutrition, since children affected by malnutrition are more likely to succumb to infectious diseases. A treatable condition, with inexpensive oral rehydration therapy, diarrhea remains a leading killer of millions of poor children worldwide. Concomitantly, increasing numbers of people are developing noninfectious illnesses (which are often very expensive to treat) due to excessive consumption of energy-dense processed foods, toxins, and pollutants associated with development. Bacteria and viruses that are resistant to conventional medical therapies have been increasing worldwide, particularly among marginalized and institutionalized populations (such as prisoners and nursing home residents), signaling a resurgence of infectious disease in more developed areas of the globe. According to the World Health Organization, food-borne illnesses continue to have a major impact even in the most developed countries, such as European member states, where epidemics still occur (World Health Organization 2010).

Food is much more than a basic need for survival and adaptation, cutting across all domains of human sociality: it is a deeply symbolic and emotional aspect of cultural identity and relationships, a pawn in the economic and political dealings of households, communities and states, and a valuable resource for wellness and healing, which is embedded within complex systems of interpretation and classification that differ dramatically among human groups (Counihan and Van Esterik 1997). Dietary choices mark the members of groups (as when pork-avoidance or vegetarianism are central to religious identities), being in a certain special state or situation (such as avoidance of alcohol when pregnant or avoidance of meat when fasting) or being in a particular kind of relationship with one another (exemplified by sharing a symbolically marked food or beverage in a religious ritual such as Shabbat or Communion).

Cross-cultural research has shown that traditional cuisines (foodways) take ample advantage of what is edible in the local environment and tend to be rich and fairly balanced in necessary nutrients and calories. Sometimes these local diets include items that have to be intensely processed (according to traditional methods, including grinding and cooking) to be made more digestible, less perishable, or remove harmful toxins. Even in environments that are very arid, such as the Arctic Circle, humans have figured out how to obtain a wide array of nutrients from foods such as roots and berries, seaweed, seal and fish. In fact the study of traditional diets indicated that there are no "essential foods" that all humans need to consume, "only essential nutrients" (Gadsby 2004). That is, we do not have to have a particular food to obtain vitamin C or magnesium or protein: a variety of sources of these will do equally well. Humans have been culturally creative in obtaining needed nutrients throughout the world, sometimes from invertebrate sources.

Every culture includes foods that are forbidden at certain times (during pregnancy, during particular illnesses, or during ritual fasting) or entirely forbidden (considered dirty, dangerous, disgusting, or inedible). Women are forbidden from eating certain foods that may harm the baby and are often encouraged to eat other foods that are beneficial. These categories are defined differently in different cultures, depending on local cultural and religious beliefs. People tend to combine traditional and recent (imported or modern) views of different foods. For example pork is considered polluting by Muslims and Jews. However, some reformed or nonobservant Jews eat pork freely nowadays. A traditional prohibition is called a *taboo* and refers to an object (or action) that should not be touched (or practiced), either because it is considered sacred or perceived as dirty, shameful, or harmful. Engaging in a taboo behavior, contact with a taboo item or ingestion of a taboo food typically brings punishment, misfortune, illness, and possibly death, usually from a supernatural source (ancestors, spirits, or God).

Mary Douglas's (1966) influential analysis of Leviticus argued that Hebrew dietary law marked certain animal foods as forbidden for the Jewish people, because they did not appear to fit neatly into preexisting classificatory schemes. Dietary laws worked to maintain symbolic borders between ritually "clean" and "unclean" objects, persons, and practices. Anomalous or improper sea creatures such as fish without scales (including shellfish) were prohibited; so were animals with split hooves that did not chew their cud (pigs) and those that chew their cud but lacked hooves (hare); those that have improper locomotion (crawlers) or too many feet were also prohibited. In addition, the body of the sacrificial animal had to be unblemished, like the body of the priest himself. Animals that were mutilated, deformed, damaged, or visibly sick in any way could not be offered, just as people who appeared "blemished" or ritually unclean were not permitted to approach the sacrificial altar (Douglas 1993). Douglas argued that cultures tend to associate danger and dirt with those things that do not fit neatly in the culture's scheme of classifications. This rule permits cows, sheep, and goats, while forbidding consumption of pigs. Each culture has different cultural classifications (which are symbolic classifications) that determine the properties, safety, or benefits of foods. In areas where humoral systems and models are used (China, India, South America) people identify foods as being hot or cold. This is not based on the spiciness or temperature properties of the food, and different cultures may consider the same food as having opposite properties and uses for health and healing.

Marvin Harris (1989 [1974]) has made a persuasive ecological–materialist argument regarding beef prohibition in India, noting that more people can be fed with agriculture than meat production. Harris has also argued that an underlying ecological reason why people in the Middle East avoid pork is that pigs are not well suited to living in arid environments, where they have to compete with humans for the same foods and become overheated, since pigs do not sweat: that is why they must roll in mud to stay cool. Meanwhile, pork is central to the culture of New Guinea people, for whom pigs represent life and wealth (Strathern and Stewart 1999). There, blood and grease are considered two humors that are necessary to health and must flow freely and be replenished in order for health to be maintained, both at the individual and the social level. People in New Guinea exchange pigs to correct social imbalances or compensate for injury and offense. A good leader "makes grease" for his community.

Anthropologists writing about the experiences of indigenous peoples have shown that colonialism, modernization (which is frequently referred to as development), and most recently globalization have had a deeply negative impact on the health, status, cultural traditions, and standard of living of native peoples (Bodley 2007;

Comaroff and Comaroff 1993; Harper 2002; Johnston 1994; Parreñas 2001). Increasingly, people are replacing local food sources and traditions with imported Western-made or Western-style items like macaroni, sodas, and potato chips, while local plant relaxants and beverages are supplanted by cigarettes and alcohol. Native modes of subsistence are threatened by political boundaries, property lines, epidemics, market forces, and industrial pollution (Ellwood 2008). All over the world, indigenous people are being heavily affected by smoking, excessive alcohol use, depression, dietary changes contributing to diabetes and obesity, and environmental pollution. Families are split apart so that parents can migrate or commute to participate in modern economic opportunities, often by working low-status and low-wage jobs and living in crowded and pestilent-infested urban areas.

The American Health Foods Movement in the Early Twentieth Century

Adherence to dietary rules continues to define cultural and religious communities and alternative lifestyles, many of which express an ecological consciousness and the desire to promote local resources and a return to "nature." Historian Michael Ackerman (2004) points out that the roots of an American health foods movement based on nutritional science goes back to 1910, when vitamin deficiencies resulting from new food processing methods were first identified. Nutritionists found that crops, animals, and humans in certain areas of the country were deficient in minerals, due to mineral-deficient soils. In the 1930s, a number of mainstream health practitioners believed that the health of Americans was harmed by processed foods, such as white flour, and began promoting alternatives available in the health food stores, including the use of vitamins and minerals. As noted in the goal statement of the American Academy of Applied Nutrition (AAAN), the movement's founders "saw themselves as conduits of information between the nutrition laboratory and the medical and dental professions" (Ackerman 2004:56). This notion of conduit of information gives vivid expression of the "flow model" of health and illness that links information, biology, and health, as discussed earlier in this chapter. Mainstream physicians and dentists critiqued the movement as promoting exaggerated claims (that all ailments are due to malnutrition) and profiting from the sale of products to a gullible public. But respectable research studies showed that millions of Americans had poor diets that left them malnourished, and there was concern that a malnourished population could not adequately defend their country in times of war, leading the Roosevelt administration to organize a vast educational campaign, provide vitamin supplements to industrial workers, and promote the enrichment of flour with three vitamins (thiamine, riboflavin, niacin) and iron (Ackerman 2004:57).

Ackerman (2004) notes that there was concern among American health foodists with preserving the natural fertility of "living soil" and the health of the environment, the impact of commercial fertilizers (robbing the soil and the cultivated plants of trace elements normally supplied by organic fertilizers and compost), the long-term effects of pesticide use, and the potential danger of artificial enrichment or supplementation of foods. Foregrounding the environmental conservation ethos that emerged in the 1960s, activists expressed concern with the disruptive effects of humans on the natural environment and opposed the fluoridation of water, viewing it as the mass use of a toxic drug to treat a preventable disease. They blamed the misapplication of technology on corporate capitalism and denounced advertising as a way to promote unhealthy consumer behaviors. However, they did not reject all new technologies as long as they did not harm the soil or alter the nutritional composition of foods. A number of health foodists were sympathetic to the movement known as "decentralism" or "distributism," which denounced the impact of modern urban industrial capitalism on people and nature, making people dependent on the government and big business. Factory work and urban consumer life were considered to be dehumanizing and unsatisfying compared to rural life and farm work, which allowed more intimacy with nature. Based on some research studies showing that stress and other individual factors may influence nutritional needs, and that additional amounts of essential nutrients may increase fitness and longevity (in rodents), some raw foodists believed that the Recommended Dietary Allowances (RDA) established in 1941 by the National Research Council were set much too low. Ackerman (2004:67) observes that, while drawing on scientific studies in nutrition, the health food movement was deeply swayed by antimodernist sentiments and motivations, and by attributing most illness and even aging to unhealthy eating, it failed to acknowledge or address the distinct needs and risks of the poor, for whom expensive health foods and supplements were not an option.

Rising Trend: Alternative Consumption Movements in the Developed World

Skipping ahead in time, it must be noted that many of the contemporary heirs of the health food movements of the nineteenth and early twentieth centuries continue to blend an environmental ethos with a critique of industrial capitalism and its patterns of food consumption. Some examples are the slow food, vegetarians, freegans, locavores, and raw foods movements. Born in Italy, the slow food movement represents a challenge to the fast-food culture and multinational corporate capitalism, along with everything that the typical fast-food chain meal symbolizes: the cheap, impersonal, rushed, processed meal that contributes to the alienation and malnutrition of millions of people and the indoctrination of new generations of consumers worldwide, while supplanting local restaurants and culinary traditions and manipulating the emotions of children by the provision of free plastic toys. On its website, the international organization describes itself as nonprofit and member-supported, "founded in 1989 to counter the rise of fast food and fast life, the disappearance of local food traditions and people's dwindling interest in the food they eat, where it comes from, how it tastes and how food choices affect the rest of the world" (SF 2011). The notion of *eco-gastronomy* conveys "a recognition of the close connections between plate and planet." The movement promotes the notion of being a *co-producer* rather than a consumer, which means taking an interest in how food is made and becoming more involved with the producers as partners. Members are part of a local *convivium*, 1,300 such chapters being in existence. Slow food (SF) has taken a politically active role in lobbying for biodiversity by promoting artisanal producers and helping them find a market for their products. In the United States, they have been lobbying for better quality foods to be available in schools. A biennial gathering of participants from all over the world, Terra Madre began in Turin in 2004 with almost 5,000 delegates representing 130 countries, bringing together cooks, scholars, food-lovers, students, and activists. The number of Terra Madre communities around the world that practice small-scale food production has surpassed 2,000 (SF 2011). Similar food movements have emerged elsewhere, such as a growing African American network that promotes healthy "soul food" in the Washington, DC, area.

While some people renounce animal products for religious reasons, many modern vegetarians and vegans choose their diets for a blend of ecological, health, humane, and spiritual reasons, pointing to the documented cruelty and animal rights abuses of factory farming, the overuse of hormones and antibiotics in industrial food production, the negative effects of saturated animal fats on cardiovascular health, the heavily polluting and energy-intensive nature of meat production and beef production in particular, and the spiritual and ethical appeal of nonviolence. Freegans aim for a zero carbon footprint by dumpster diving and other strategies of avoiding the purchasing of foods or the payment of rent, to minimize their environmental impact and retract from the capitalist cycle of spending and consumption (explore freegan. info for a more detailed online account). Locavores aim to promote sustainability by eating more local foods, which are believed to be less contaminated than imports and do not need to be transported across hundreds or thousands of miles, thus reducing the consumption of fossil fuels. Other movements and designs for sustainability have emerged under the name of *permaculture*, spearheaded by David Holmgren, Bill Mollison, Geoff Lawton, and other visionaries. Permaculture espouses the view of human life as enmeshed in sustaining relationships with Earth's mineral, plant, and animal forces. It holds that humans need to return to growing their own food, even in urban areas, and working with the natural features of the land, blending modern science with traditional knowledge to create sustainable designs for living and food production, such as sustainable forest gardens and urban gardens, in order to heal our relationship to the Earth. A closely related cultural phenomenon, "urban homesteading" emerged as an alternative lifestyle and movement for self-sufficiency, eco-consciousness, and economic de-growth: decreasing environmental impact through reducing consumption of manufactured and industrially produced goods and foods, use of secondhand goods, urban gardening, egg and manure production, use of energy-efficient designs and technologies, reduction of nonrenewable energy use, and increased use of alternative energy sources such as biodiesel (Urbanhomestead. org 2010).

Humoral Medical Traditions, Foods, and Herbs

Local healing knowledge and wisdom exist in every culture, having been transmitted primarily through oral traditions. Ancient rock art points to the probable existence of rituals involving hallucinogenic and shamanic experiences more than 35,000 years ago (Clottes and Lewis-Williams 1998). In the course of human evolution, stone tools and the management of fire enabled the ancestors of today's human populations to expand their food base and geographical range, enhance sociability and protection from predators, and modify certain foods to make them more digestible and safer by cutting, grinding, and cooking. Archaeological and ethnographic evidence suggests that indigenous knowledge and use of psychoactive substances such as cacti, vines, mushrooms, and herbs probably date back several millennia and are intimately connected with healing in small-scale societies. Recognized by humans long before written records, the value of foods and herbs for health maintenance and treating illnesses is well documented in the oldest existing medical treatises in Mesopotamia, Egypt, and Babylon, as well as Sanskrit medical treatises from the second millennium B.C.E. Roots of elaborate traditional healing practices of the Central Andean "Health Axis," stretching from Ecuador to Bolivia, extend back to archaeological records of the Moche period (100–800 C.E.) and comprise hundreds of plant remedies, including foods and spices that have recognized health benefits, such as the now-globally marketed "superfood" *Maca* (Bussman and Sharon 2006).

Nina Etkin's (2006) book *Edible Medicines: An Ethnopharmacology of Food* takes a biocultural or ecological perspective on food and foodways, drawing attention to the medicinal, organoleptic, and pharmacologic qualities and potential of foodstuffs. Her ambitious and wide-ranging work demonstrates that the reductionist paradigm of biomedicine—which considers disease apart from the person and the social context, divides the body into component parts, prioritizes crisis management over prevention, and looks for a specific cause for every ailment—is currently giving way to a more humanistic model of therapeutics that is amply supported by cutting-edge research on the biochemistry and human ecology of foods, revealing their key role in wellness and healing, both in minimally processed form and as the latest "pharmafoods" (Etkin 2006:81).

The notion that food is medicine is not entirely new to Western medicine; it lies historically at the very origin of biomedicine. In classical Greece, around 400 B.C.E., authors of the Hippocratic Corpus affirmed that diseases had natural causes, rather than magico-religious ones, and promoted the notion that opposites cure opposites (later identified by the term *allopathy*) and declared that food is the best medicine. Much of the Corpus is devoted to dietary prescriptions, with an emphasis that illness is best prevented by a diverse diet adapted to individual needs, such as age and health status. More food should be consumed in winter and spring, when the digestive tract is "hottest"; barley soup, vinegar and water, and honey and water are among the many recommended remedies for epidemics; and many foods were cataloged for their particular health benefits (Etkin 2006:47). The dietary prescriptions were related with the doctrine of the four humors—earth, air, fire, and water—natural forces that had to be kept in proper balance and proportion for health to be maintained or restored. These forces were connected with bodily fluids, times of day, seasons, stages of life, and personality traits, as shown:

- earth: mucous (phlegm); night; winter; senescence; phlegmatic temperament
- air: black bile (melancholy); evening; autumn; late middle age; melancholic
- water: blood (sanguine); morning; spring; childhood/youth; sanguinary
- fire: yellow bile (choler); mid-day; summer; adulthood; choleric temperament

Hippocrates was followed by Discorides (ca. 40–80 C.E.) and Galen (ca. 120–200 C.E.). Discorides created *De Materia Medica*, a five-volume work that cataloged 1,000 remedies, mostly botanical, with 4,740 medicinal uses, including recommendations such as picked olives to aid digestion. Galen developed the Hippocratic approach into a more rigorous therapeutic system, where foods were on a hot–cold and wet–dry axis and used in precise food/medicine combinations for particular illnesses, developed through extensive experimentation. Illness was considered and treated as part of the person and the person was viewed as an integral part of nature and coterminous with it (Etkin 2006:48–50).

A close examination of Hippocratic and Galenic diagnostic and therapies shows them to be empirical, reasoned, flexible, and pragmatic. Not surprisingly, their influence extended throughout the ancient world, being translated into Arabic and elaborated on by Arabic scholars, particularly Avicenna (980–1037 C.E.), and becoming the basis for Greco-Islamic medicine or Unani Tibb, which continues to play a significant role in many countries today, including Malaysia and Pakistan. In the sixteenth and seventeenth centuries, the pharmacopoeias of Europe were expanded as a result of contact with the New World, the origin of medicines such as curare (a muscle relaxant), ipecac (an emetic), quinine (from the Chinchona tree), cocoa (a stimulant), and coca (a sedative), as well as chili peppers, corn, and potatoes, which transformed the cuisines and economies of Europe (Etkin 2006:58, 89–92). Aztecs used chili peppers for dental problems, sore throat, asthma, and cough. Recently, they have become some of the popular ingredients in today's latest "phytoceuticals" (Etkin 2006:92).

Along with providing sustenance and medicine, foods have constituted a valuable means of gaining favor and control, promoting harmonious relations, and displaying success, both economically and politically. Food is an important medium of exchange and pacification with the human world as well as the spirit world.

From pressures to replace native foods with nutritionally inferior cash crops and monocropping to the prized packets of imported coffee used to secure favors under communism, and the global expansion of nutrient-poor but calorie-dense fast foods based almost entirely on corn, food is an arena of manipulation, exploitation, and contestation (Bodley 2007). The demand for provision of certain foods in certain quantities has been integral to many relationships of loyalty or domination, exemplified by the payment of tribute in the form of staple crops practiced during the times of imperial conquest and colonial occupation worldwide. For example, the province of Wallachia, now a part of Romania, was required to pay their tribute to the Ottoman Empire in wheat, which caused the local peasantry to depend increasingly on corn for survival. The profound connection between food and cultural identity is illustrated in the fact that rice functions as metaphor for the Japanese self and a key element in rituals, whereas blue corn is at the heart of the Hopi creation myth and a metaphor for the Hopi self: the Creator gave the Hopi the smallest yet hardiest corn to signify their endurance. Symbols and metaphors are often grounded in bodily experiences, building cognitive and emotional bridges between the biological and the social world. When we examine the role of foods in health and illness, we must recognize that the use and value of particular foods for particular purposes results from a combination of biological and environmental factors together with historical, political, economic, and symbolic elements that characterize a particular time and place.

Organoleptic qualities of foods are those qualities that are perceived through the sense organs. *Sight* alone can attract or repel: the bright and shiny appearance of a firm apple or the bruised and withered surface of an overripe fruit. The perception of *flavor* is derived from taste and smell together. Olfactory nerves tie into portions of the brain that are responsible for memory and emotion, suggesting the complex linkages between taste, smell, and the personal and cultural meanings of food (Etkin 2006:32). *Textures* of foods vary in their cultural significance: whereas a green bean cooked to mushiness recalls the comfort of home to an American southerner, a crisp green bean that offers resistance, followed by juiciness, constitutes an aim of Chinese cooking (Etkin 2006:33). The sense of *hearing* also plays a part in food-related experiences: the blend of crunch and squish of the granola yogurt, the fizzy drink, or the crackle of food cooking in a pan can stir up vivid images, desires, and associations (Etkin 2006:33).

Nina Etkin (2006:31) notes that childhood is marked by a preference for sweet and salty tastes, which are associated with safe foods, whereas bitter taste is often a marker for toxicity. Bitterness commonly signals that a substance has medicinal properties, indicating the presence of *alkaloids*: the family of chemicals that includes quinine and coffee. Tastes such as bitter, sour, and astringent are common criteria for selecting medicine across cultures. The *doctrine of signatures* describes a principle of organization found in many cultures, whereby likeness signals therapeutic or ritual efficacy. Thus, yellow fruit are commonly used for treatment of liver ailments (which may lead to jaundice, signaled by the yellowing of the eyes). Plants that ooze white liquid or flowers with white petals may be used to stimulate lactation. Those with red flowers or leaves may be used for bleeding. Vines with heart-shaped leaves may be used for ailments of the heart. Plants with many flowers or fruit and animals that produce multiple offspring are used by the Hausa of Niger to promote fertility (Etkin 2006:39). Avoidance of foods may be dictated by tradition as a remedy for illness, according to humoral principles that divide foods in hot/cold, wet/dry categories and tend to vary widely across cultures. Among the Hausa people, food plants that impart a gelatinous quality to soups must be avoided if one has flu or backaches believed to result from an accumulation of phlegm (Etkin 2006:40). Individual aversions to particular foods can develop from unpleasant experiences, pointing to the manifold interactions among the cultural and the biodynamic involvements of food.

Spices have had enormous geopolitical significance, being traded in India and Mesopotamia for more than two millennia. Current pharmacological research on spices demonstrates that they have antimicrobial properties, which explains why the use of spices would provide a survival benefit, being more widely used in hot climates, where food is more likely to breed bacteria, and more abundant in meat dishes than vegetable dishes (Etkin 2006:98–9). Abundant research has been taking place on the ample health benefits of fermented foods, which are used in nearly all cultures. In Western countries yogurts and kefirs, as well as capsules and powders containing *probiotics* have become a popular health food supplement, being credited with improving digestion and replenishing the "good bacteria" in the intestinal tract after antibiotic treatment. The immune system is dependent on the proper functioning of the gut and the presence of beneficial gut flora. This is acquired at birth and during the days portpartum from the mother and can be maintained in proper balance as long as one is healthy and well nourished. Unfortunately, the intestinal balance is commonly disrupted by biomedical treatment, including hospital birth.

Scientific research on the composition and effects of probiotics and fermented foods is now being carried out worldwide. Fermentation destroys some undesirable elements; foods become more digestible; new flavors and textures are generated; the need for cooking and fuel is diminished (Etkin 2006:112). In addition, fermented foods have been shown to have diverse antimicrobial and anticancer effects. Native cultures worldwide rely heavily on fermentation in their cuisines. For example, Nigerians consume more than thirty fermented foods. Four primary nutrient-rich fermented foods are used to strengthen women postpartum and during weaning, and for newly circumcised boys. The most important condiment in Nigeria, the pungent *daddawa* is a concentrated soup base and flavoring made of seeds that are inedible when raw (Etkin 2006:128–9).

There is tremendous biodiversity in bacterial flora among geographic regions and producers. Native strains of microorganisms that come from local soil and air are responsible for the unique flavors of products. In the United States and Europe, recent food hygiene laws mandating pasteurizaton and limiting the sale of unpasteurized foods have caused hardship for small producers and elicited protests from consumers and advocates for the health benefits of raw and unpasteurized foods. There is a trend in the United States among urban sophisticates and seekers of more natural foods toward the consumption of unpasteurized "artisanal" cheeses, a statement of class distinction as well as a form of protest against large-scale production and standardization. Drawing on her fieldwork among raw-milk cheese makers in Vermont, Heather Paxson (2008:17) coined the term *post-pasteurian cultures* to describe the grass-roots efforts to reclaim microbiological diversity in a culture that has been permeated by fear of germs. She argues for the need to consider *microbiopolitics*: "the creation of categories of microscopic biological agents; the anthropocentric evaluation of such agents; and the elaboration of appropriate human behaviors vis-à-vis microorganisms engaged in infection, inoculation, and digestion."

Case Study: ELTA Universitate—Natural Foods, Anesthesia, and Social Renewal

To highlight the complexities and entanglements of food, health, tradition, and politics, I offer my own account of the Romanian healing movement ELTA Universitate, based on my 1998 fieldwork on alternative healing in Romania. ELTA emerged in the wake of the collapse of communism as a call to physical rejuvenation, spiritual awakening, and social transformation. While critiquing modern consumption practices, ELTA promotes a raw, lacto-vegetarian, locally grown diet, believed to be essential for spiritual growth, social healing, and the evolution of humanity. Echoing Marx's critiques of capitalism and religion, ELTA members affirm that people are sickened and *anesthetized* by contemporary life, and its participants believe their regimen cures cancer and diabetes, enhancing sexuality and longevity. Because ELTA denounces the routine pasteurization of milk as morbidity-inducing, its views on living healthfully contrast with the public health guidelines of the EU. During the group's periodic three-day retreats, ELTA's charismatic leader, Ion, speaks to participants about goals, spiritual awakening, astrology, journaling, sexuality, mental hygiene, food production and preparation, technology, and the meaning of money. The group produces and sells uncooked dry bread denoted as "mana," said to have rejuvenating and healing properties, but the most advanced stage of their diet is liquid, using unpasteurized milk and local honey. Through their website, ELTA encourages communication and self-knowledge through a variety of methods and techniques, including regular retreats as it denounces mainstream views on health maintenance and promotion (Eltauniversitate.ro 2011).

Some outsiders might perceive Eltists as belonging to a "cult," but this anthropologist would disagree, since the group's emphasis on individual quest, self-knowledge, and personal agency does not fit the common definition of cults. Markers such as rigorous diet, strong convictions, a powerful sense of community, a preference for white or light color clothing, and very long hair set the members of ELTA apart socially. At the same time, Eltists' efforts to expose the larger society to their ideas and knowledge through food exhibits and menu delivery to subscribers (many of whom are chronically ill) serve to keep them connected and interacting with many other social segments and groups. ELTA members believe that the task of informing others of the physical and spiritual benefits of the raw-foods diet is a social and spiritual duty. They view their task as one of spreading light (knowledge) and opening up a path for the salvation of society. From the ELTA perspective, the "anesthesia" and limitations that are induced by modern materialism and consumerism are certain to lead only to physical and spiritual decay.

Prominent anthropologists like Jean Comaroff (1985) and René Devisch (1993) have written about the "disease of modernity" and the importance of healing practices in cases of rapid social transformation. Devisch (1993) observed that healing movements appear to be most central when people feel lost, dislocated, or in times of accelerated social change. Definite similarities exist between ELTA and other utopian communal groups or "other-worldly" sects, as John R. Hall (1979) described them. Like many other-worldly groups, ELTA is characterized by a critical view of society at large, a demanding regimen (dietary restrictions and work), the existence of a charismatic leader, a community of goods, messianic ideals, and an apocalyptic interpretation of current history, which is expected to come to an end, to be replaced by a community of the awakened. The ELTA community strives to create its own, higher-level society and also to be a haven from the surrounding world of consumption, ignorance, and greed. Yet ELTA does not strive to isolate itself completely from the rest of society, as millenarian groups typically do. Hall has pointed out that most other-worldly sects practice religiously inspired communism. Interestingly, even though ELTA discourse firmly rejects dialectic materialism and communist definitions of the person, echoes of communist ideology have come to the fore on occasion. One such example was the following statement by Ion, the group's charismatic leader: "Communism is not possible if people are not healthy and their minds whole." Ion also affirmed that the formula "to each according to need" should apply when distributing resources within ELTA, both among individuals and among the smaller branches of ELTA found in various cities.

One of ELTA's young physicians said in a lecture that "ELTA is creating a society, a civilization," and compared ELTA with a zygote or a functional embryo, connected through the umbilical cord to the rest of society and to the world. The same young doctor stated that medicine will be the way to salvation for society, because "the

Idea: Modernity also brought possible trade offs.

instinct of pain is the only one greater than the instinct of money." He insisted that, to have an impact on others, one must work primarily on oneself: "If you do not save yourselves, the rest of society cannot be saved either. Do not make the patient become dependent upon you. One must heal oneself." He then carried the organic analogy even further, adding: "We live in an amniotic fluid. Living in this embryo you receive light. You must believe more strongly in light than in money. You are all doctors, your own doctors." ELTA explicitly strives to restore agency to the individual and rebuild the sense of self, as well as establish new values and alternate ways of relating to others. Unlike some spiritual or religious groups who seek converts but otherwise minimize their interactions with the outside world, healing-oriented movements tend to place high value on social involvement and community, despite the occasionally acknowledged risk of being negatively influenced by harmful vibrations or energies.

Clearly, as an alternative healing movement, ELTA is a "total phenomenon," to paraphrase Marcel Mauss (1990 [1950, 1925]). Its discourse cuts across all social domains and represents a concerted effort at carving out new individual and social identities, restructuring power relations, and establishing a new value system in the context of the postcommunist transition. Sontag (1990), Crandon-Malamud (1991), Comaroff (1985), and other scholars have pointed out that the language of healing is effectively used to challenge hegemonies and renegotiate new meanings and relationships in both personal and collective spheres. Verdery (1991) discussed the centralization of meanings and the attempted disablement of older significances that characterized the impact of communism on culture. She wrote: "Leaders trying to install a new symbolic order aim to destroy or absorb into the political apparatus alternative orders and alternative meanings not yet bent to a new will. Wars are declared on cultural accumulations of an older era . . ., as new accumulations are slowly amassed. The possibility of different claims and justifications, of a different construction of reality, that these older forms contain cannot be permitted to flourish" (Verdery 1991:97).

A key aspect of the communist agenda for progress was to transform citizens into proper workers and docile bodies, as well as to enforce a uniformity of thoughts and practices, which was particularly effective in the area of state-controlled health care. Foucault's (1994 [1973]) work well established the centrality of the body as an object of domination and a key site for the dialectic of power and knowledge, speaking of the descriptive act of medical science as "a seizure of being": an active way of shaping perception and creating knowledge. Indeed, post-1989 medical pluralism seems to have begun as an effort to reclaim the symbolic domains of the self, body, health, and illness, which had been completely controlled by the political apparatus of socialism prior to December 1989. Yet healing has also become an incisive challenge to the expanding hegemony of consumer culture as well as being a systematic deconstruction of communist legacies, ideologies, and structures, some of which are still present.

In many ways postsocialist healing movements are akin to millenarian revitalization movements in their efforts to reclaim a lost or primordial state (of health, moral rectitude, and sociocultural well-being), their quasi-nationalistic ethos, their voiced suspicion of money and profit, and their criticism of and opposition to Western individualism and materialism. From this perspective, ELTA's emphasis on the consumption of pure, raw, unprocessed food and their advocacy of a "natural" way of life for the purpose of revitalizing self and society can be interpreted as a reaction to the alienation brought on by the "shock therapy" of transition and rapid encroachment of Western-style modernity. David Sutton (2001:75) argues that the synesthetic experience of eating can play a key role in one's efforts to return to "wholeness"—an older, truer, and more meaningful way of life. Sutton (2001:77) wrote that for Greek migrants experiencing a longing for "home" and a sense of disjunction, "food is essential to counter tendencies toward fragmentation of experience." Furthermore, the act of eating food "from home" carries the implication of an imagined community, in addition to the real communities that are generated and sustained through shared consumption (Sutton 2001:84).

Lucian Boia (1998:14), a contemporary Romanian historian, points out that "the original communist project aimed at the liberation of man, of *alienated* man, as Marx himself said. Man was to rediscover himself, to become free. All constraints eventually had to disappear," including the state itself. The family too was to be transformed into a free and more flexible union, as a result of the achievement of equality between the sexes, Boia writes (1998:14). He adds: "The millennial, thus anarchical, roots of Marxism appear in a very clear light. The accent falls more in the individual than upon the social body, with the observation that, once social contradictions would be resolved, the incongruity individual–society would not exist anymore. Individual and society become one" (Boia 1998:14). Nevertheless, the contradictions did not go away. As Boia indicates, the deepening contradictions led to the metamorphosis of man's liberation into the gruesome enslavement of totalitarianism.

It is valuable to note similarities between Marx's *alienation* and the ELTA concept of "anesthesia." This medical metaphor of mass disempowerment effectively appropriates Marx's argument and imagery. But whereas for Marx, the opiate of the masses was religion, for Eltists the drug of domination is food, the state of mass anesthesia being the direct result of indiscriminate consumption and restricted access to information. Both perspectives emphasize that the generalized powerlessness is a result of ignorance and manipulation, and both postulate that for the creation of a higher social order, the individual must be radically transformed and his power and agency restored, an ideal exemplified by the "new man" of communism.

Reclaiming production, which was instrumental to Marx's vision, was also a significant aspect in ELTA members' vision of their future society. In speaking of mass production and the routinization of labor, Ion said that repetition is usually an anticreative act and thus gives rise to "sin," a state of lowered vibrations that appears at the moment of multiplication, mass production, and standardization. In one lecture, Ion said to group members that by purchasing raw materials from intermediary merchants "you become the slaves of dealers who are at the middle of the road and take advantage of both you and the producers," echoing the deeply ingrained distrust of middlemen and markets that was a staple of communist mentality, and which continues to be widespread in Romania and the former Soviet Empire. In support of production, he also asserted that both produce and milk can become charged with low vibrations from certain intermediaries. Ion argued that barter is not primitive but, rather, natural, and that markets as intermediaries entail additional costs, such as the retailer's own mark-up, as well as sales tax. In his view, there is a "natural price" for things, which is not generally what one can get in the marketplace. "Money too is matter, a kind of barter, albeit a more allegorical, metaphorical, symbolical one," he said. A small community does not need money, but it is a necessary evil in interactions with the larger world, for acquiring "such necessities as computers, cars, apartments and cellular phones." Referring to money as *curentul verde* ("the green current"), Ion insisted that, without tapping into this force, ELTA could not progress or reach its full potential as an engine for social change.

Prominent ELTA members repeatedly expressed their dislike of money as a social instrument and their negative view of its effects on people and society. Using the term *curentul verde* may appear like an effort to redeem it, by pointing out its importance in linking people together and transferring influence and resources. Yet having an alternate name for money parallels the traditional Romanian practice of having multiple alternate names for the Devil or Satan. According to folklorist Ivan Evseev (1994), popular Romanian mythology has as many as eighty-two alternate names for the Devil (*Diavolul* or *Dracul*), such as The Drooling One (*Bălosul*). Orthodox Romanians commonly believe that one should not even speak the name of "the unclean one," for that makes his presence manifest, giving him power over the person who spoke it. At the same time, Evseev (1994:54) points out that popular mythology attributes to *Dracul* trickster-like qualities, like intelligence, craftiness, and playfulness. In Romanian folklore *Dracul* is a necessary evil, as illustrated in the popular saying "Make yourself brothers with the Devil until you cross the bridge" (Evseev 1994:54). A similar perspective applies to the ELTA view of money—a necessary evil that, if co-opted or tamed, can be of great utility.

The etymology of the word *drac* goes back to the Greek or Latin terms for dragon, meaning "big snake," considered a protective spirit of the home; it is only with the influence of Christianity, Evseev (1994:54) notes, that the attributes of the Devil have been transferred on it. *Curentul verde* seems to invoke this protective mythical dragon, along with connotations of fertility and vitality, while the avoidance of the term *money* echoes folk beliefs in the contagion and augmentation of evil through the spoken word. These beliefs are continuous with local Romanian traditions, as well as being present in ELTA's formal discourse on the power of words, the elemental nature of information, and the deep interrelation of the physical and mental dimensions of the universe, as not naming is an effective way of removing oneself from an undesirable influence and thereby restricting its power.

There is a need to rethink money and to question its moral value and implications in the face of changing social and political circumstances. ELTA discourse speaks of the need to "tap the green current" and thus makes an explicit effort to appropriate its symbolic power, to apprehend and domesticate "its energy," and to rethink "its morality" along new coordinates, shaping it into something compatible with ELTA's own personal, ethical, and spiritual framework of social development and self-actualization. Lucian Stratan, a young physician who was one of the leading ELTA speakers at the time of my fieldwork, argued passionately against the quest for money in the practice of medicine and accused medical practitioners of culpability in the creation of the "planetary disaster" and "generalized pathology" we are currently witnessing. According to Stratan (1997:9), "the purely materialist education that medical doctors receive has dehumanized medicine, turning it into a craft, creating robots that repair mechanically other robots." Modern medical care is a futile battle as long as doctors advocate the consumption of meat or processed foods; as long as they disregard the role of the mind, behavior, and education in the etiology and treatment of disease; and as long as they fail to fulfill their responsibilities as teachers and metaphysicians.

Health is dependent on thinking, understanding, and education, according to ELTA Universitate. Illness and death result from ignorance and disregard for the principles of life, when people do not care for themselves by cultivating mental, nutritional, and sexual hygiene. Having established these three empirical aspects of self-care, the person becomes not only healthier but also able to benefit fully from the study of metaphysics and to engage in discovering one's highest purpose. The Absolute Divinity created only Light and Life, whereas Death and Disease are outcomes of human civilization, and the cumulative effect of existential errors committed again and again.

Of Information and the Triadic Approach

The emphasis on information is a key element in the ELTA worldview. It is also central to many other contemporary healing movements, the human person being described simultaneously as an energetic system and an informational system. Conceiving of information as an elemental aspect of the universe is not a new trend in Romanian thinking. The prominent Romanian physician and anthropologist Victor Săhleanu in 1972 dedicated an entire book, *The Science and Philosophy of Information*, to this topic. In this work he provided a thorough review of previous concepts and theories of information and put forth an interpretation of all biological life as having three forms: substance, energy, and information (Săhleanu 1972). This view is still widespread among Romanian intellectuals and healers.

The triadic model of the universe runs deeply through Romanian culture and tradition, owing partly to the Orthodox Christian emphasis on the Trinity, although it undoubtedly has deep pre-Christian roots. The number 3, like the numbers 9 and 7, are of paramount importance in the fairy tales, myths, and legends of the Indo-European world. Many of these certainly predate Christianity and continue to play a major role in the imagination of all modern descendants of Indo-European peoples. ELTA, as well as other alternative health movements in contemporary Romania, holds firmly to the view that most universal processes have three aspects, forms, or stages, and that any approach or model should always have a triadic structure, rather than a dual one. Many old Romanian folk tales have the dualisms present in the form of good daughter/bad daughter, prince/monster, rooster/hen, friend/enemy, young/old, true/false. However, just as many stories privilege the number three: three daughters, sons or daughters-in-law, three magical encounters, three trials. The third is predictably the most fortunate. A strong cultural preference for triads challenges the classic structuralist generalizations about human cognition as being predicated chiefly on oppositions. The "traditional Romanian outlook" does not favor oppositions, but triads, as cognitive tools.

The "law of the triad" is explicitly described by ELTA's leader Ion as a *method*. In order for a process to be "dynamic and real," one must identify three components, and these three elements must be "premeditated." According to Ion, "duality is a linguistic and sensory confusion," an illusion of appearance or perception as exemplified by the duality between man and woman. ELTA's formulation of the fourth universal law of *Kybalion* affirms that all things have two polarities, all polarities and paradoxes can be reconciled, and all truths are ultimately but half-truths. On the surface, each element of a triad may be "dual," as there is always an oscillation, a vibration, Ion has noted. However, on a more profound level, each element of a triad indexes yet another triad.

According to bioenergy healer Soranu, who was also a member of ELTA, the quintessential triad is the divine Trinity, composed of the Father, Son, and Spirit. Soranu affirmed that the Holy Trinity exists within us, like a "sphere" or a "code." We were created from these "conscious particles." The "mental" aspect of the person refers to one's capacity for thought. Everything is spirit—everything is mental. Man creates through thought-forms, which remain linked to their creator, Soranu said. Creation is thus a separation of the creator from thought-forms. However, God is the Word, the Word is God, and in the Word there continues to exist the spiritual form of the Creator. Soranu pointed out that numbers are also spirits, like letters and words. The number 1 is the unity, the divine; 2 is duality, or the physical world; and 3 is the Holy Trinity, the triad, representing the human person and God. "God self-created as a triad," Soranu added. The person is represented by the number 10, symbolizing both unity and infinity. Through the practice of self-knowledge we return to ourselves, which is the return of the son to the father. The son has been transformed— "the prodigal son." In Soranu's words, the spiritualization of the body constitutes this return. The body longs for perfection, just like the soul. Thus, numbers, bodies, and spirit are interconnected.

Energy, Dowsing, and Information

The diversity of healing options and approaches I encountered in Romania in 1998 was simply astounding. I spoke with homeopaths and acupuncturists formally trained as medical doctors, physicists, and engineers who practiced radiesthesia (a type of dowsing) and reiki, and a scholar who studied energy "auras" as possible sources of diagnostic information. I learned of many herbalists who had become well known for the curative preparations they invented and who had their own private offices and clinics; some of them held chemistry or biology degrees, others were based in local knowledge, and some were even said to be self-taught. I was informed of many interesting healing practices and practitioners by my Romanian Fulbright advisor Dr. Ioan Oprescu: a female psychiatrist who used pyramids in psychotherapy, a controversial medical doctor with visionary abilities, and an opera singer turned healer who used sounds and colors together with a knowledge of chakras and body meridians. However, it was not practically possible to pursue every such opportunity or to investigate all of the approaches that aroused my anthropological curiosity.

During my fieldwork I attended a national alternative medicine conference together with Dr. Cornelia Guja, a biophysicist from Bucharest's Francisc I. Rainer Anthropology Institute. Dr. Guja was a guest of honor at the conference. She has been conducting biomedical research using an *electrograph* device and a technique akin to Kirilian photography: images of the hands and feet taken after a brief electrical discharge were used to identify correspondences between the patient's health status and the aura-like electrical patterns captured on film, classifiable as positive (anodic) and negative (cathodic) electrical discharges. Most of the conference events took place at the former Culture House of the Unions in Arad, a large neoclassical building with a spacious auditorium. In the entrance lobby of the conference hall there was a multitude of display tables with herbal products, as well as books, cookbooks, booklets, newsletters, and magazines on each and every topic in alternative healing, from yoga, reiki, and auras to the sites of religious pilgrimages and healing icons of Romania. Dr. Guja had her own collection of beautifully illustrated color brochures on display, in Romanian and English translations: *The Human Being: A Biointerface between Microcosm and Macrocosm, a Hypothesis That Can Be Experimented*

Today (No. 1, 1996) and *The Human Being: A Biointerface of Archetypal Communication* (No. 2, 1997).

The booklets discussed the electrical nature of the universe and of life and the basic, archetypal structures of nature as postulated by Dr. Guja. One such fundamental structure is an ovoid, coined by Dr. Guja as the *integrom*, which is represented by the egg, the atom, the solar system, or the human body and its auras. Another structure emphasized in the brochures is a branching tree, an "archetypal form of communication" and a building block of branch-like networks. Like the ovoid archetype, tree structures and networks are found everywhere in nature: tree roots, lightning, spider webs, human hands, skeletons, vascular or river systems, neural tissue, fractals, and human made "artificial networks." Dr. Guja's model of the person as a relational being integrated into an unceasing flow of universal communication, her electrographic images, and her concept of the *integrom* were perceived by conference organizers and participants as a scientific acknowledgment of the aura model of the person, a central and uncontested aspect of Romania's alternative healing universe. From the various presentations at the conference, it became evident that backing healing practices and models with scientific theorizing, experimentation, and validation is an important concern for those seeking mainstream legitimacy for alternative therapies.

Many of the papers at the conference used scientific language and cited experimental results to support alternative therapies. Papers written by university-trained scientists documented laboratory experiments that employed info-energy techniques also known as *radiestezie* (dowsing) for various purposes: to increase the efficiency of certain chemical reactions between a plant and a symbiotic bacterium, to modify the hardness of a dental alloy, to inhibit the growth of the polio virus and enhance the fitness of cell cultures, or to alleviate pain. Radiesthesia uses a modified dowsing rod to obtain information from the "Universal bank" or network and manipulates bioenergy using hand motions and the power of the practitioner's mind. Other talks touched on the challenges of quantifying the results of various alternative therapies and the value of documenting the results of working with children from a distance ("distal therapy"). Most frequently, as one of the presenters acknowledged, the result of the therapeutic act is a "synergistic effect" of allopathic medicine, unconventional therapies, and the placebo effect, which cannot be eliminated except in cases of small children who are treated from a distance without being told. A large number of conference papers emphasized the spiritual, divine, or magical alongside moral, personal, and social implications of the different therapies.

Imre Lázár (2006) paints an equally vibrant image of the new pluralism that characterizes postsocialist societies in his exploration of the reinvention of the Táltos tradition, folk healers who use dowsing, prayer, energy, light, and "spirit surgery" to diagnose and heal a variety of discomforts, often very effectively.

He dubs them "neoshamans," noting that they practice an ancient form of ritual and spiritual healing, which is not the same as that of the original Táltos tradition but yet represents an ancient way that is known all over the world (Lázár 2006:40–1). Lázár notes a first step in becoming a Táltos is being initiated in dowsing, which enhances the healer's connection with the inner self, as well as allowing access to information and knowledge from outside the self. The healers interpret the act of dowsing as aligning oneself with the divine will. In the process of dowsing and energy work, the Táltos operates in "astral" space, using his "astral glove": the palm chakra. The practitioners seem to induce a light state of trance in the patient and have been known to produce powerful experiences of healing or remission in their patients for conditions not treatable by biomedical means. Lázár compares the community created between healers and patients with Turner's anti-structure, noting the communal element of the therapy in the case of a seventy-year-old woman with an inoperable brain tumor. The Táltos healer who performed "spirit surgery" also involved her son in the treatment, initiating him into sending her energy. Her partial paralysis resolved, her status improved, and she remained symptom-free two years later (Lázár 2006:46).

Despite lack of scientific confirmation that it works better than chance, dowsing continues to be a popular practice, and its popularity in the field of alternative healing has grown tremendously in Eastern Europe, where many folk healers use it to diagnose their patients and measure the subtle aura energy of different organs or parts of the body. In my Romanian fieldwork, I observed radiesthesia practitioners use dowsing in combination to prayer, bioenergy, massage therapy, and the application of infrared radiation along with other physical therapies, within an explicit context of Orthodox Christian faith. Dowsing has been used for millennia throughout the world, primarily for finding water sources under the ground, thus the name of "water witching," but it has also been used for finding objects or persons, or gaining insight into problems, sometimes from a great distance. Although scientifically dowsing has not been demonstrated to work consistently better than chance and some consider it fraud, in their research Vogt and Hyman (2000 [1959]:163) found no basis for this view: in every case that they encountered, "the diviner was an honest man of recognized integrity," a part-time practitioner, who would more often than not perform the service free of charge to help his neighbors, rather than for commercial gain. The authors recognized dowsing as a form of *magical divination*, a ritual activity of gaining knowledge about hidden or future events, and that persists in both rural and urban areas of the United States "because there are potent psychological and social reasons for it":

There is undoubtedly a deep and enduring human propensity to engage in divination that will translate the unknowable into knowable, the uncertainties into certainties, and this divination is engaged in by curious scientists and by rural water diviners alike in their search for knowledge of what lies beneath the surface of the ground. (Vogt and Hyman 2000 [1959]:192)

It is a satisfying and meaningful practice that entails a "cognitive embodied field of practical mastery" and the unequivocal perception of a "hidden reality," Lázár suggests (2006:42), noting that such a method of knowing is comparable to Mauss's (1973) notion of bodily technique, introduced in the 1930s. Laying the foundation for Bourdieu's fruitful reformulation of the concept *habitus* decades later, Mauss first introduced the term *habitus* to describe socially inculcated demeanors and practical orientations, such as elements of physical posture or movement, a learned art of using the human body in the realm of everyday life, acquired through imitation, noting that cultural techniques are *effective* and *traditional*, while they may be at the same time magical and religious (Mauss 1973:73–5).

Galina Lindquist (2006) provided a nuanced, lively, and provocative account of magical healing in Russia, drawing on her experiential fieldwork with a variety of nonbiomedical healers in 1999. She shared Arthur Kleinman's (1995) dissatisfaction with the interpretive approach in medical anthropology—the ways in which oppressive power differentials played out when an anthropologist imposed his or her interpretation on another person's experience of suffering, as when a medical professional imposes a clinical diagnosis upon the patient. Drawing on social phenomenology and Kleinman's call for the use of "experience-near categories," Lindquist's (2006:11) analytical approach involved shifting her goal to discerning "what is at stake" for her informants: instead of interpreting people, following their own processes of interpretation along with them. She revealed how cultural creativity expressed through magic enabled healers and their patients to transform their experience of suffering in productive and efficacious ways. Vivacious biomedical doctor and bioenergy therapist Nina S. attributed independent agency to her healing hands (Lindquist 2006:149), as did the Maya bonesetters described by Servando Hinojosa (2002) in Guatemala—"the hands know" what to do.

From the art of listening to a patient, to the use of an egg or their hands to cleanse away negative energies (also popular throughout Central and South America), to psychodynamic treatment that helps clients in the management of emotions and relationships, or the use of traditional spells for every conceivable purpose, Russian practitioners of magical rituals often interpreted their actions and successes as changing the "bio-energy-information field of the patient" (Lindquist 2006:160). Lindquist concluded that magical practices and the archaic language of spells depended on local relational dynamics of power and sociality, deep historical roots, and strong social bonds in order to provide a social poetics of hope and survival, an intersubjective interpretation of suffering, and the ability to persist through difficult circumstances.

QUESTIONS FOR CLASS DISCUSSION

1. Free-list familiar food avoidances and prohibitions. How are they justified and enforced? Can you see biological, psychological, social, or ecological benefits?
2. Think about the effects of seasons and weather conditions on health. Do you see seasonal patterns of change in your own health? If so, how do you explain them?
3. Ask students to write down four "healthy" and four "unhealthy" foods they consume often. What are their justifications? What factors are involved in making these decisions?
4. How does health information available online influence the way you care for yourself and your family when you have an illness or disease? Do you mention it to your doctors?
5. Interview each other about plants that your family or friends use as therapies or tonics when someone is ill. Where do these practices originate? How have they survived?

QUESTIONS FOR ESSAY WRITING

1. Write a persuasive argument for or against the consumption of unpasteurized milk and milk products while acknowledging the best arguments that oppose your own view.
2. Research and write an essay about the cultural origins, symbolic associations, ecological impact, and economic costs and benefits of something that you consume regularly (coffee, sugar, cotton, etc.). How does this habitual consumption impact your health or others? Try to point out social and political inequalities involved, locally or globally.
3. Come up with five key ingredients to robust mind–body health, in your own view, and reflect on how they are shaped by individual or social/economic/political circumstances.
4. Select one herbal therapy that has been growing in popularity (such as consumption of fish oils) and write an essay teasing out its history of use and social entanglements.
5. Identify a plant that has recently emerged as a popular health supplement or product (such as açai, hoodia, maca, or turmeric) and explore its traditional cultural context of use.

SUGGESTED READINGS

Gumpert, David E. (2009), *The Raw Milk Revolution*. White River Junction, VT: Chelsea Green Publishing Company.
Lipp, Frank J. (1996), *Herbalism (Healing and Harmony, Symbolism, Ritual, and Folklore Traditions of East and West)*. New York: Little, Brown and Company.
Sutton, David E. (2001), *Remembrance of Repasts: An Anthropology of Food and Memory*. New York: Berg.

RECOMMENDED FILMS

Darwin's Nightmare (2004), by Hubert Sauper.
The Dreamers of Arnhem Land (2005), by Christopher Walker; Australian aborigine elders sustainably harvest and market traditional resources on ancestral lands.
The Future of Food (2004), by Deborah Koons Garcia.
The Shaman's Apprentice (2001), by Mark Plotkin.
Waste = Food (2007), by Ron van Hattum.

INTERNET RESOURCES

Chocolate, Cheese, Meat and Sugar: Physically Addictive Foods (40 min.), lecture by Neal Barnard MD, founder of Physicians Committee for Responsible Medicine, http://video.google.com/videoplay?docid=-3058533428492266222#docid=-3214100593069532942.

The Future of Food: What Every Person Should Know. Massachusetts School of Law Educational Forum, Kurt Olson's discussion with filmmaker Deborah Koons Garcia, http://www.youtube.com/watch?v=m6rEQqOemlk.

Hippocrates: *On Ancient Medicine,* written 400 B.C.E., http://classics.mit.edu/Hippocrates/ancimed.html.

Marion Nestle lecture, "What to Eat: Personal Responsibility or Social Responsibility?" http://www.youtube.com/watch?v=iRLA7THDIDw.

The Weston A. Price Foundation for Wise Traditions in Food, Farming and the Healing Arts, http://www.westonaprice.org/.

–3–

Spirit, Consciousness, and Trance

Whether we think of it as soul, mind, or spirit, human consciousness has played an important role in healing, variously embedded in local cultural worlds and widely acknowledged cross-culturally, since the most ancient times. A universal life principle that distinguishes what is alive from what is dead and that transcends the death of the body is referenced as early as 1500–1000 B.C.E. in the Vedas, the sacred scriptures of India: the Sanskrit concept of *atman*, a core concept in Hindu philosophy. In pre-Christian Europe, the Greek *psyche* and the Latin *anima* described a similar entity. Early Indo-European traditions identified soul with breath and viewed it as an integral part of the natural and physical world, an individual entity responsible for one's inner reality and a variety of cognitive functions, emotions, desires, and moral qualities; but later on, when soul was relegated to theology, some of these qualities became associated with "the mind" (Olafson 2010). As in Vedic India and classical Greece, where contemplation, restraint, and diet were all used in the search for knowledge and self-transformation, a number of early Christians took refuge in the Middle Eastern deserts to seek spiritual transformation and direct experience of the divine. The lives and words of the Desert Fathers were recorded in the *Philokalia*, which remains to this day an important source of knowledge and revelation in Orthodox Christianity, particularly in Eastern Orthodox monasticism.

The understanding that a spirit realm that interacts with the visible realm exists throughout the natural world has been well documented by numerous anthropologists in societies worldwide. While lacking the formality of written records and philosophical treatises, in small-scale societies there is a widespread notion that an invisible, universal source of power (which could be described as *spirit*) permeates the natural world. One of the earliest anthropologists, Sir Edward Burnett Tylor, created a hierarchical typology of religious forms in his book *Primitive Culture* reflecting the colonial and Judeo-Christian bias that founders of anthropology shared in the nineteenth and early twentieth centuries. Tylor (2009 [1903]) described *animism* as the simplest form of religion, "the belief in Spiritual Beings," thereby coining one of the earliest and most influential and enduring anthropological concepts. At the turn of the century, the prolific scholar Sir James George Frazer (2000 [1922]) believed that magic emerged before religion as a form of pseudo-science, but despite this condescending bias, he made a valuable and lasting contribution by identifying the two relevant principles of magical action: the principle of similarity that underlies *sympathetic magic*, that like things influence one another, and the principle of contagion that underlies *contagious magic*, that things that are in contact will remain connected and continue to interact even after they have become separated. These ideas are found as readily in the great religions as in the great medical traditions.

Tambiah (1968) drew on Malinowski, Leach, and Bloch as he asserted the instrumental role of language in magical endeavors, exemplified by the ancient and widespread notion of word as deed. Actions and words together make up ritual and magical power. This vital force of words is captured vividly in the very first biblical statement "In the Beginning was the Word," or references to Jesus as "the Word" in the Christian tradition, or the words or sentences called *mantra* in the Sanskrit tradition, which have great transformative power when repeated over and over in meditation—but variations of this idea are found in many cultures. Tambiah (1979) has argued that there is no conflict between the rationality of Western science and the truth of magical acts, as they are grounded in radically different premises. The basic operation of science is doubt and it requires proof, whereas the basic operation of ritual is trust and it relies on powers of persuasion, felicity, and normativity: if ritual actions and words are correctly performed, the magical act possesses "illocutionary force." This efficacy is manifested at times when words and gestures such as "with this ring I thee wed" accomplish the change of a person (as well as changing a couple and the relationship of two families) from single to married.

Susan Greenwood (2009) is a practitioner of magic as well as an anthropologist. She notes that science was born from the blending of natural philosophy with sympathetic magic, the latter being co-opted into the experimental approach. Since the seventeenth century, however, science has considered matter to be separate from mind. Magical consciousness emphasizes participation, analogy, emotion, and the language of *mythos,* whereas science emphasizes causality, logic, objective assessment, and the language of *logos,* notes Greenwood (2009:145). She advocates a dynamic model of consciousness: a web that includes both magical and scientific modes of knowing, an integrative consciousness operating through mental maps, guided by imagination and metaphor in perceiving, apprehending, and creating patterns. Greenwood (2009:151) draws on philosopher Gregory Bateson's concept of *abduction*: a type of reasoning that organizes information through metaphor. Magic has its rightful place to reclaim.

The notion that some peoples or religions are less evolved cognitively than others has been strongly and repeatedly disproven since the now bygone era when the term "primitive" was used by anthropologists, art historians, psychologists, biologists, and other scholars, while chauvinists with xenophobic and eugenic agendas upheld hierarchical schemes of step-by-step cultural development and social evolution. Genetic evidence based on mitochondrial DNA indicates that, while human groups are distinctively adapted (biologically and culturally) to particular ecological niches, all humans on earth today are related via mitochondrial DNA to an ancestral African female *homo sapiens* dating back around two hundred millennia B.C.E.;

genetic research also seems to indicate that a most recent common ancestor of all humans alive today lived much more recently. Oddly perhaps, since it contradicts our common sense, genomic research shows that, despite the commonality of dark skin, native Melanesians are less genetically similar to native Africans than the latter to native French. Thus, visible racial differences and markers that have been privileged historically as means of classification of "biological races" obscure more major similarities and differences at the genetic and molecular level, which more accurately reflect genetic closeness/distance among ethnic and geographical populations. The arbitrariness of racial classification and its political and social manipulation have been amply documented in history and anthropology in the twentieth century. Irish and Jews were once considered another race in the American South. In the Caribbean and South American countries, more distinct racially mixed categories exist than we recognize in the United States. In countries that have the reputation of being homogeneous ethnically, deep internal divisions exist among minorities and majorities who have different statuses and rights: this is the case of the socially stigmatized group the Burakumin in Japan (Lie 2004) or the influential Uighur (Muslim Chinese) in the Xinjiang province of China, who are allowed more than one child and other benefits as a result of their minority status (Gladney 1996).

The most recent genetic research indicate that modern humans are more closely interrelated and interbred across racial boundaries than formerly anticipated. Therefore, there are no "primitives" on earth in the evolutionary sense. Whether they possess written records of their histories and their accumulated knowledge or not, all living humans and human groups, are equally distant from a recent ancestor, thus equally "evolved." Adding to the mystery of commonalities and universals, ethnographic work reveals that there is no such thing as "primitive religion": native mythologies and religious traditions, while predominantly animistic, have been shown to be sophisticated and imaginative, on par with the most complex theistic traditions known. Common themes and symbols span the world's religions and rituals: the existence of mythical heroes that die and come back to life (Maya, Apache, Christianity), cunning tricksters (Anansi the spider in African tales, Coyote among Native Americans, Rabbit in the American South, the Fox in Europe), variations on the Cinderella story (China, Korean, English, Scottish, Native American), and enormous floods (just about everywhere on Earth, even in the driest or most elevated places). Myths, religions, and rituals reflect and codify particular historical and ecological realities, exploring universal human themes and concerns, imbuing life and suffering with meaning, providing comfort, hope, and cohesion to communities as well as transmitting cherished life lessons, social norms, and a variety of cognitive benefits for survival.

Ritual practices and religious movements have long been demonstrated to have a variety of functions, including social (affirming and sometimes challenging the social order, according to Durkheim and Turner), emotional (relieving anxiety about the unknown, according to Malinowski), cognitive (creating meaning and coherence out of difficult life/death events and experiences, according to Lévi-Strauss and Geertz), and ecological or environmental (fostering a sustainable relationship through traditions such as food taboos, which are responsive to environmental features and balance, according to Roy Rappaport (1968), Marvin Harris (1989 [1974]), and G. Reichel-Dolmatoff (1976), among others). In the 1930s Malinowski (1935) showed that magical practices and special incantations of the Trobriand islanders of the Pacific worked to alleviate fears of the uncontrollable in their endeavors, while being combined with ample practical knowledge of gardening: magic *and* science were thus employed together to promote human ends and foster well-being. Evans-Pritchard (1976 [1937]) addressed the ubiquity of witchcraft among the Azande people of north-central Africa, showing that they regularly blended pragmatic interpretations of events (such as the barn fell down because it was old and rotten) with witchcraft beliefs. For the Azande, every misfortune also had a supernatural cause and explanation for why it afflicted a certain person at a certain time. The term "primitive" fell into disrepute and the notion that magical beliefs are irrational superstitions has been amply contested, with ethnographic evidence showing the richness and complexity of indigenous traditions and explanations. While myth and magic are still used in popular speech to mean false or irrational ideas and actions about the world or the origin and nature of events (particularly those of rural and indigenous people and less developed societies), modern studies of religious behavior have demonstrated that all cultures (simple or complex) comprise some "magical" elements and practices, which are experientially and culturally persuasive, relevant, and authentic, thus *real* in their social and lived power and effects, such as Gmelch's (1978) famous essay on "baseball magic."

Since the 1960s, anthropologists such as Marcel Mauss, Claude Lévi-Strauss, Victor Turner, Mary Douglas, Clifford Geertz, Stanley Tambiah, and Thomas Csordas have shown less concern with ranking or categorizing of religious phenomena than with exploring the ways in which cultural symbols, categories, meanings, and rituals enabled and shaped key experiences, understandings, and embodiments of the self, the sacred, and the supernatural in various places and times. Such scholars have made numerous contributions and played instrumental roles in shaping the contemporary understanding of ritual and magical practices, including rituals of healing, as culturally contingent performances with true *efficacy* that is derived from cognitive, symbolic, rhetorical interactions and experiences. Many ritual actions and therapies may not be "proven to work" by the standards of science (although they have been shown to induce evident changes, physical and mental) but possess ritual or spiritual efficacy and power; thus they may be efficacious in their transformative impact on the consciousness of participants and the social context. In a classic anthropological example, in the Pacific Islands native peoples experience a diffuse and impersonal spiritual substance called *mana*, which may be present in all things, particularly living things, and which concentrates in persons of high social standing, such as members and families of the upper classes and powerful leaders, who can share its power and benefits with others. *Mana* can grow through generosity and warfare, among various means, or be diminished through arrogance, anger, and selfish deeds. At the very beginning of the twentieth century, Mauss (1972) described the multi-factorial and paradoxical qualities of this vital force as being akin to a fourth spatial dimension of awareness, invisibly underscoring the consciousness of Pacific Islanders in the same fundamental way as Euclidian principles underlie Western understanding of space. *Mana* is pervasive, yet cumulative, divisible, yet whole, impersonal, yet personal, while manifesting "automatic efficacy" (Mauss 1972).

In his famous essay "The Effectiveness of Symbols," Lévi-Strauss (1963) described the power of a South American healer's chant of a mythical journey in facilitating a very difficult birth. In her influential work *Purity and Danger*, Mary Douglas (1966) provided elegant arguments showing that entities that do not fit neatly in established cultural classifications schemes tend to generate ambivalence, revulsion, fear, or prohibitions and deftly pointed to the body as a natural symbol for a broad range of experiences and theories. Turner's (1969) research on ritual symbols and pilgrimage asserted their deeply transformative potentialities as catalysts and arenas for social communion and change, not simply the preservation and transmission of mythical knowledge and cultural values. He explored at length the similarity between religious movements and rituals of transition, described by Arnold van Gennep (1873–1957). A central notion in van Gennep's proposed three-part model of rituals is the passage from one life stage to another through a transitional phase, charged with symbolism, which is often associated with healing and renewal. Turner (1969:95) focused on this phase of liminality and the persons experiencing it as deeply ambiguous, "neither here not there," or "betwixt and between," being characterized by the formation of *communitas:* a distinctive homogenizing community in the ritual process, which has the potential to change or renew society (Pandian 1991:122). Applying van Gennep's model to the study of illnesses as rites of passage has generated valuable insights into the experiences of severe illness as a transformative journey, especially for chronic or life-threatening conditions, where sufferers experience a death-like loss of their former selves and their former lives, as well as the inception of a new life stage and a transformed sense of self (Frank 2002).

Clifford Geertz (1973) pioneered the interpretive turn in anthropology by affirming that cultures are texts: symbolic systems to be felt, read, and interpreted while "looking over the native's shoulder." Geertz also played a defining role by celebrating the complexity and the ethnographic richness of "thick description" in elucidating the symbolic system of a culture in action. Placing yourself in the middle of ethnographic action to absorb the meanings and effects of symbols through all the senses has been instrumental for modern scholars of shamanistic healing and other types of spiritual healing, as it was for Geertz in describing the Balinese cockfight that he fled, frightened, to seek shelter. Since then, many anthropologists have taken experiential participation and ontological and epistemological engagement with their subjects to new dimensions, some becoming apprentices and advocates of shamans, herbalists, mediums, and sorcerers, others earning doctoral degrees in medicine, chiropractic, nursing, and public health. Marcus and Fischer (1986) described the contemporary moment in anthropology as an experimental moment that promises to broaden the relevance of ethnography. Classic norms of participant-observation that aimed for objectivity having been demasked as fictions many times in the past thirty years, anthropologists have used themselves as data-gathering instruments in arenas such as divination, magic, and healing (Tedlock 2005; Lindquist 2006; Greenwood 2009).

In carrying out my own fieldwork in Romania in 1997–1998, I tried to take for granted as little as possible and endeavored to attend with sincerity, experiential participation, and suspended judgment on my informants' accounts, their physical and emotional expressions, and the context of the ethnographic moment. My model for the ethnographic encounter and its subsequent recounting and analysis was that of a dialogical exploration of epistemologies and modes of engagement focused on individual actors, joined with as much experiential identification and immersion (a bit like "going native") as I was able to achieve. My experiential and physical involvement with particular alternative healing approaches was inspiring and essential to the production of my ethnographic account, although it sometimes felt like a simulacrum of "true participation"—a theatrical performance. While recording and analyzing the fieldwork data, I endeavored to keep in mind the heteroglossic nature of cultural forms and to explore potential meanings, together with the production of meanings. Although "experience always far exceeds its description or narrativization," as Byron Good affirms (1994:39), narrative forms of representation are a primary means of access to others' experiences and "have a complex relationship to experience." Focusing on narratives and discourses of illness and healing, strategies of persuasion, and the performances of speakers, I wanted to elucidate how various social, economic, and political factors played into the production of meaning, knowledge, and authority. I also sought to gain insight into how discursive and narrative acts were situated within the moral landscapes of my informants and what they revealed about the historical underpinnings of their moral worlds.

Altered States, Bodies, and Souls

With regard to medicine, the premises of Western science have historically become materialistic to an extreme, to the extent to which psychiatry and mental health generally have increasingly become brain-centered and brain-based, particularly in the United States where recent decades have witnessed a pervasive and progressive shift to a therapeutic culture of medication over talk therapy and behavioral interventions. Like physical illness, anxieties, moods, and obsessions are increasingly located in biological and biochemical structures and pathways. Arguably, in this tradition the self and the personality have increasingly become viewed as biochemical side effects of the genes' and organism's fight for survival and reproduction. In contrast, traditional healers and ritual healing traditions such as shamanism, witchcraft, pilgrimage, and spiritual healing frame the self as sacred and focus on the creation and maintenance of "sacred human identity" (Pandian 1991). In his exploration of religious healing among Charismatic Catholics, Thomas Csordas (1997 [1994]) showed how prophetic speech achieves transformative power in this growing community. Ironically, such seemingly opposing views of self and personhood have begun to converge increasingly in recent scholarship: a growing body of ground-breaking work that bridges neuroscientific data and psychoneuroimmunology with first-person accounts of healing experiences (as both witnesses and participants) written by anthropologists interested in phenomenological approaches to healing and consciousness, many of whom have amply documented their own involvement with healing and ritual methodologies. Psychoneuroimmunology is a branch of biomedical sciences that explores' manifold (and yet poorly understood) mutual interactions between mental states or stimuli, the nervous system, and the immune system, to identify the physiological and biochemical pathways that account for the complex interconnections.

In small-scale indigenous societies, ritual specialists traditionally journeyed to unseen worlds through dreams and visions to gain insights into human problems and heal suffering, retrieving lost, stolen, or dislocated souls and soul fragments. They plead, wrestle, and negotiate with disgruntled ancestors and nonhuman beings that inhabit less tangible experiential dimensions. Referred to by anthropologists as *shamans*, from a Siberian language term for such indigenous practitioners, these local leaders and healers purposefully enter altered states of consciousness to communicate with the spirit world, in order to bring healing and wisdom to their communities and the afflicted. Shamans are traditionally both revered and feared as possessors of ample traditional knowledge of the natural and the supernatural worlds, from herbal medicines to magical incantations for divining and redressing the causes of illness and misfortune. This powerful knowledge is transmitted orally and through apprenticeship from generation to generation, but much of it can also be gained through dreams and visions, intuitive experience, and practical hands-on experimentation, including trial and error.

According to the earliest art found on rock and cave walls, altered states of consciousness may have played an important ritual role in human cultures going back 40,000–100,000 years. Until recently (the past two hundred years) human existence on Earth has been characterized primarily by community- and family-centered practices of healing, as spiritual needs, emotional needs, social needs, and physical needs all played a role in illness, therapy, and recovery. With the rise of the Enlightenment and scientific rationalism in Western Europe, the notion that mind and body are separate entities and that the mind deserved primacy over the body took on new and influential dimensions and achieved great social prominence and status, captured in philosopher René Descartes's famous reflection, "I think, therefore I am." Embodying the cultural sentiment of the modern era, rather than Descartes's singular insight, this polarization of the mental and the physical dimensions of experience became known as "Cartesian dualism" and found ample expression in modern Western science and medicine, as the tendency to view spiritual, mental, emotional, and physical awareness and well-being as separate domains. This perspective is reflected and embedded in the structures of Western civilizations, such as the separation of church and state, the separation of pastoral counseling, psychoanalysis, psychiatry, and social work, or the separation of mental health from physical health in most Western health systems, as well as the modern Western cultural emphasis on the individuality and independence, rather than collectivity and interdependence, which bear greater value and significance in non-Western cultures.

At the level of daily practice, diverse local cultural traditions do not embrace the same sharp distinctions between and within mind, soul, and the physical body as people do in developed Western societies today, nor do they acknowledge the same parts or subdivisions of these realms or categories, just as cultures do not make the same anatomical or physiological distinctions when looking at the organization of the human body. While it is well known and accepted that "beauty is in the eye of the beholder," it is much less known that local notions of anatomy or the map of the soul might also be in "the eye" of the beholder, where eyesight has been trained by cultural lenses to notice and appreciate some things over others. Thus, the Maya of Guatemala speak of and palpate an abdominal organ called the *tipte*, involved in childbirth (Jordan 1992); Hindu ethnomedicine practitioners and many different types of contemporary energy healers (including yoga and reiki practitioners) seek to stimulate energy centers called *chakras*, seven wheel-like vortices located along the spine, from the base of the top of the head; at the same time, Traditional Chinese Medicine (TCM) practitioners work along multiple energy points and meridians, feeling and interpreting hundreds of bodily messages and connections, visible or hidden, many of which have never been perceived or employed (diagnostically or therapeutically) in Western varieties of scientific medicine. Kuriyama (2002) eloquently recalled the ancient poetic language used to convey the manifold haptic variations of clinically relevant pulses: sunken, rough, slippery, or floating, in the words of Li Shizhen, "like a subtle breeze blowing across the down of a bird's back" (Kuriyama 2002:98). Scholars of TCM have documented national efforts toward standardization alongside the real-world plurality and diversity of TCM in China, in time and in space, along with its many transformations through globalization as it has adapted to fit the expectations of local clienteles (Hsu 1999; Scheid 2002). While it is generally perceived to be slow-acting when compared to biomedicine, Chinese medicine is perceived as fast-acting and "advanced" medicine in Tanzania, where Chinese doctors commonly provide treatments that integrate Chinese and Western medicines (Hsu 2002:307).

Similar diversity exists when it comes to conceptualization of the soul. In the fifth century B.C.E., bringing into focus fuzzy and material notions of the soul that permeated the centuries that preceded him, Socrates asserted the immortality of the soul

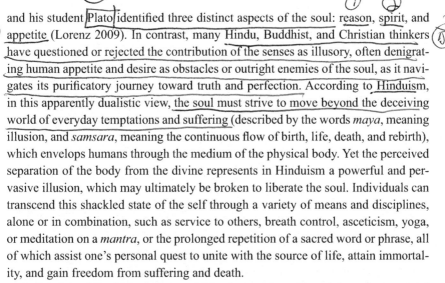

and his student Plato identified three distinct aspects of the soul: reason, spirit, and appetite (Lorenz 2009). In contrast, many Hindu, Buddhist, and Christian thinkers have questioned or rejected the contribution of the senses as illusory, often denigrating human appetite and desire as obstacles or outright enemies of the soul, as it navigates its purificatory journey toward truth and perfection. According to Hinduism, in this apparently dualistic view, the soul must strive to move beyond the deceiving world of everyday temptations and suffering (described by the words *maya*, meaning illusion, and *samsara*, meaning the continuous flow of birth, life, death, and rebirth), which envelops humans through the medium of the physical body. Yet the perceived separation of the body from the divine represents in Hinduism a powerful and pervasive illusion, which may ultimately be broken to liberate the soul. Individuals can transcend this shackled state of the self through a variety of means and disciplines, alone or in combination, such as service to others, breath control, asceticism, yoga, or meditation on a *mantra*, or the prolonged repetition of a sacred word or phrase, all of which assist one's personal quest to unite with the source of life, attain immortality, and gain freedom from suffering and death.

In Hindu and Buddhist cultures, deification can be achieved through sequential cycles of death and rebirth, which are partially influenced but not necessarily determined by one's spiritual efforts and everyday behaviors in the current life. The notion of *karma* refers to large-scale cause and effect cycles, explaining one's current state (including wealth, social status, health, or suffering) in terms of a benefit or burden of previous deeds, whether carried out in this life or a former one. It may seem ironic that while predicated on the search for absolute bliss, this worldview can lead to a mortification (renunciation) of the body and greater acceptance or tolerance of suffering (whether one's own or that of others) as inevitable, necessary, or even formative human experiences, a perspective that may impede efforts to change society or to improve on structural—social and political—sources of poverty, suffering, and inequality. Thus, the social division of Hindu society into a fairly rigid system of social castes, with specific social roles that make some of the castes so ritually and socially impure as to be "untouchable" (the group that slaughters animals or the one that burns dead bodies) reflects in some ways a fatalistic view: that one must accept his or her lot in life and hope for a better birth in the future. However, tremendous diversity exists in local interpretations, practices, and traditions of Hinduism and Buddhism in different countries and communities, some of which (such as tantric schools of Tibetan Buddhism and Yoga) openly and richly celebrate the body and all the senses as doorways to enlightenment, healing, and blissful union with the divine.

Haitian vodoun (or voodoo) practitioners, most of whom are practicing Catholics, speak of the existence of not one but two souls, *ti-bon-ange* (the little angel, one's individual soul, which may be harmed or alienated during trance and through witchcraft) and *gros-bon-ange* (the big angel, or the shared life force); these souls interact in sleep, dreams, wakefulness, ritual trance, or death with the interests and the powers of the *loa* (or *lwa*): various meddling, quirky, demanding, often moody spirits located in between the realm of the one supreme God, *Bon Dieu*, and the mundane world of humans. With distinctive, quirky personalities like those of the Hindu deities and the Greek gods of Olympus, the *Loa* embody diverse qualities of popular West African deities and many have Catholic saint counterparts, acquired during centuries of slavery, when propitiating African gods was forbidden and slaves were forcefully Christianized. Both *Loa* and ancestors bestow blessings as well as illness or misfortune. Thus, despite the ill reputation of voodoo perpetuated in the media, many rituals of vodoun are primarily healing rituals, lubricating or redressing relationships with the spirit world, the natural world, and the social world, while expressing and addressing concerns and conflicts found in the world of the living, particularly sickness, grief, and loss.

Some cultures speak of multiple souls or soul parts that can be lost, stolen, or fragmented, intentionally or inadvertently, with dire consequences for persons and their families. Traditionally, the Hmong people of Southeast Asia, many of whom have become refugees in the United States since the 1970s, have practiced an animistic religion, the oldest form of religious worldview, which has characterized most small-scale societies until very recently. Widespread among indigenous people in the Americas, Africa, and Asia, *animism* can be described as the belief that spirit(ual) substance or power imbues all aspects of nature: animals, trees, mountains, rocks, rivers, and places. This view expresses a kinship and intimacy with the natural world, which contrasts with the view of human dominance over nature that is espoused in the Abrahamic religions (Judaism, Christianity, and Islam). Often, animistic cultures also believe in reincarnation or propitiate departed ancestors' spirits, which continue to influence the living; this is the case with indigeous or tribal religions of China and Japan and the indigenous religions of Africa, which are now widely blended with Islam, Catholicism, and many other Christian denominations (Baptist, Pentecostal, etc.). Like many Native Americans, numarous Hmong have become Christian in the United States and are now experiencing painful conflict between their traditional cultural views and their new Christian beliefs.

According to Anne Fadiman (1997) traditional Hmong speak of multiple souls, ranging from one to thirty-two, while considering the "life-soul" to be the one most implicated in illness and healing. Souls of ancestors must be beckoned and honored to be born again in the same family; babies' souls, having a tendency to trail off in wonder of beautiful sights and sounds, must be fastened to babies' bodies through naming rituals and strings tied around their wrists; animal sacrifices are used to feed the souls of an ill person or the souls of ancestors and spirits that may be causing trouble for the living, including sickness; ritual healers called *txiv neeb* must negotiate with spirits for the well-being of their people. The concern with the soul's safety is so great that Hmong people often refuse procedures that are thought to endanger it, such as general anesthesia.

When Murphy Halliburton (2009) went to India to study the experience and treatment of mental illness in Kerala (South India), he expected to find "unique constellations of somatic idioms, forms of expression that offered an alternative to the modern, cosmopolitan, Western tendency to express distress in psychological idioms," but instead he found that his informants' accounts of their experiences involving states such as anxiety, sleeplessness, anger, and hallucinations, spoke chiefly about their *manas* (a Sanskrit-derived term for mind), *bodham* (consciousness), *ormma* (memory), or *atman* (the intangible self). At the same time, Halliburton (2009:153) notes that mind and body are not opposed in Kerala to the same extent that they are polarized in Western mind–body dualism: in his view, *mana* or mind exhibited a material, embodied quality that would make it closer to the body than to pure consciousness; at the same time, the patients he interviewed seemed to share an experiential orientation that involved many fine distinctions and significant concern with *other* states of consciousness, such as *bodham* and *ormma*. In Kerala, English terms of "psychological" distress are used alongside Sanskrit-derived terms in the local language, Malayalam, reflecting a blending of therapeutic options and multiplicity of interpretations at work.

In recent decades, concern with the spirit, the mind, and the emotions in confronting illness has reemerged in the arena of Western discourses on health and healing, as exemplified in the work of spirituality-oriented physicians such as Deepak Chopra, Bernie Siegel, and Andrew Weil, and in the fact that medical schools in the United States and other biomedically dominated countries have begun to offer courses on relaxation, stress-relief, and yoga as well as cultural competency courses that encourage health professionals to address and respond to their patients' emotional and spiritual needs, not just their physical needs (CU School of Medicine 2011). Increasingly, clinical evidence (CU School of Medicine 2011) corroborates the fact that, while they alleviate stress, regular relaxation, behavioral therapy, and support groups can extend lives and greatly improve the quality of life of those with severe or chronic illness (such as cardiac and cancer patients) and their families. In the insightful and moving article "Hospital as Temple," P. Leguit (2004), a medical doctor practicing in the Netherlands, glances back nostalgically at the long history of temple-based healing in the Middle East and European antiquity, and then describes his personal journey in caring for cancer patients. Leguit was struggling with feeling drained and discouraged by the death of patients, as well as becoming uneasy with referring patients with recurrences (assessed as likely to die soon) for further chemotherapy and radiation of unlikely benefit, probable to cause more harm than good. The author was strengthened and inspired by Bernie Siegel's (1990 [1986]) book *Love, Medicine and Miracles* to begin caring for patients in a different way, which included welcoming them to regular sessions with a cup of tea and offering time when they could freely draw and tell their stories. Leguit also participated in meditation classes.

This change of attitude and "bedside manner" may seem slight or superficial, but it engendered a transformative experience for both patients and caregiver: the patients felt better and coped better with an adverse course of their condition (even though half died eventually), while the doctor felt energized and regained an enthusiasm for practicing medicine. At the same time, Leguit (2004:30) describes a frustrating experience when he was kept from lighting a candle for a dying patient due to hospital guidelines. In this and many other firsthand accounts by medical professionals, there is a call to recognize medicine as a humanistic endeavor and the human experience of sickness as a complex web of influences, a biocultural phenomenon, to be approached from a variety of interdisciplinary experiences. Leguit concludes that outcomes and satisfaction may be improved by acknowledging both patients' and caregivers' spiritual needs, along with the fundamental need for trust and relationship to caregivers and family members. In a growing number of U.S. hospitals, shamans of the Hmong (Southeast Asian) and the Navajo (native North American of the Southwest) and other nonallopathic healers are now being welcomed to comfort and assist members of their cultural group alongside medical staff, as long as they respect hospital guidelines and recommendations for action.

Much anthropological research has been devoted to exploring the nature and the boundaries of minds and bodies as they are experienced and described in different cultures and the changes in these concepts and experiences across history within the so-called Western world, which itself includes a broad diversity of interpretations or traditions: the classical Latin precept *mens sana in corpore sano* (healthy mind in a healthy body), Orthodox Christian mysticism and monasticism, scientific materialism, Sufi Islam, Mormonism, Jehovah's Witnesses, New Orleans voodoo, or eclectic forms of New Age spirituality, to name only a few. It has been firmly established with the use of ethnographic evidence and anthropological reflection that cultural practices and beliefs shape the way people view and experience the self—where it begins and ends; whether the body, the mind, and the soul are perceived as separable, singular, or homogeneous entities; how they are structured and interrelated; the nature and role of relationships in configuring self and group identity; and the role of body, mind, and spirit in religion and ritual. It has also been shown that biases (ontological, phenomenological, ethical, and epistemological) rooted in Western philosophy, history, and cultural practices have shaped the work and interpretations of anthropologists and other observers of cultures.

The end of the second millennium did not trigger many newsworthy natural or supernatural end-of-the-world dramas, nor did Y2K cause cyberuniversal collapse. But it was characterized by a veritable flurry of research and writing at the intersections of consciousness, cognition, behavior, and the rapidly changing field of neuroscience, a heady blend of biochemistry, physiology, and psychology with novel advancements in imaging technology. Functional magnetic resonance imaging and positron-emission tomographic scanning have made it possible to visualize various parts of the brain during various activities, whether practicing yoga, performing jazz, solving mathematical puzzles, or watching television. This new information is then integrated with existing knowledge on how injuries, epilepsy, language, moods, or medications influence brain function or chemistry. Scholars and scientists from various fields have been intrigued about the possibility of discovering which areas or functions of the brain may be involved in creativity and religion. Some scientists argue that neural mechanisms associated with spiritual experiences may have occurred as mere side effects of evolutionary changes, driven by mammal and early hominid struggles for survival, while others use molecular biology and brain physiology and the universality of human religious experiences as evidence of God (Snyder 2008). The conflation of biochemistry and religion has recently leapt so far as to postulate the existence of a "spirit molecule"—Rick Strassman's (2000) name for DMT or N-dimethyltryptamine, a substance involved in the psychopharmacology of serotonin, found in human bodies and some plants. It is deeply ironic that some natural scientists are claiming spirituality for molecules at the very same time as cutting-edge social scientists are turning to phenomenology and "sensual scholarship" to argue for a re-embodiment of the mind, a re-cognition and re-valuation of the role and centrality of the sensual in all aspects of lived experience (further explored in chapter 4). Medical anthropologists, health professionals, and patients (acting as consumers of trends and services) now seek formal and practical recognition that mind and body are not experientially or culturally distinct or separable entities, that they are not clearly bounded or delineated the same way in all cultures, and that it is difficult if not impossible as well as undesirable to fully disentangle them in the pursuit of health, in the experience of illness, or in the practice of healing.

Because of its overwhelming emphasis on material and mechanical aspects of human health and illness, the limitations of biomedicine in satisfying the needs of patients and families have been widely discussed and documented: the ever-increasing costs of biomedical treatments; time limitations; expanding conceptual, linguistic, and social gaps between patient and provider; common-but-deadly procedural risks and intrusions; and the way bodies are objectified and divided (Foucault 1994 [1973]; Illich 1976; Scheper-Hughes and Lock 1987; Jordan 1992; Martin 2001; Rapp 2000). As anthropologists have amply documented, choices that people make and the categories used to describe bodily states and discomforts are formulated in response to local needs and environments, being inextricably bound up with social, economic, *Choice* and political values, moral judgments, and specific cultural and historical circumstances (Young 1982; Crandon-Malamud 1991; Comaroff and Comaroff 1993; Masquelier 2001). Choices are rarely neutral socially or politically, in that people usually seek to explain and redress perceived imbalances beyond biological function. Libbet Crandon-Malamud wrote in her book on Bolivia, *From the Fat of Our Souls*, that "if differential use of these medical resources stems from their [i.e., the individuals'] efforts to constantly negotiate new meanings of identities and restructure social relationships in order to gain access to resources, the logic behind the process of choice can be delineated" (Crandon-Malamud 1991:31). Choices made in caring for individual or family health are not simply personal, but political: they are charged action-statements-ciphers that on closer scrutiny deliver complex critiques of local and global processes and power relations, tools in the existential struggle to grasp, interpret, and grapple with changing demands of one's social, economic, and political environment. In this sense, the quest for alternatives is a life call and act of freedom, a power-privileged state that begins with the care for the self (Foucault 1997 [1984]).

Shamanic Consciousness and Symbolic Healing

As far back as the nineteenth century, anthropologists (including Frazer, Tylor, Boas, Malinowski, and Mauss) have provided evidence that humans everywhere have complex religious traditions and practices, and elaborate myths about the origins of the cosmos, animals and plants, human diversity, valuable skills, and powerful knowledge. Native people on all continents are documented to have out-of-the-ordinary experiences of invisible (but often sensible) yet powerful forces, powers, qualities, or beings, as well as traditional practices for communicating and interacting with such forces, commonly described by Western observers as "supernatural forces" or "spirits," except for the fact that they are very much part of everyday life and embedded in the natural world, as experienced in small-scale societies. In some cultures, such as the Ju/'hoansi or !Kung bushmen of the Kalahari, lengthy healing rituals take place, when men experience a state of altered consciousness as they dance, accompanied by the singing and clapping of the women. Anthropologists have richly documented the vibrant healing rituals of these native foragers of sub-Saharan Africa (Marshall Thomas 1989 [1958]; Katz 1982; Lee 2003). "Boiling energy" is generated by men who dance for many hours, then shared with others by laying hands on members of the band who need strength or healing. Some men experience a deep and potentially dangerous transformation of consciousness referred to as "half death."

In small-scale societies of Mongolian herders, Inuit hunters, or Guatemalan villagers, a man or a woman performs the authoritative role of ritual specialist, regularly journeying into other realms of experience to communicate with ancestors, animal spirits, and forces of nature, bringing them powerful knowledge and healing (Tedlock 2005). Practices used to achieve experiential transformation that allows communication with non-ordinary dimensions of reality have been described by Eliade (2004 [1951]) as "techniques of ecstasy." Bourguignon's (1968) cross-cultural analysis of these states, traditionally called "trance" states, showed them to be nearly universal yet highly variable across cultures, being subject to local contexts, myths, environments, and interpretations. Historically, these experiences are also documented across large-scale religions and fringe religious movements, described as ecstatic, gnostic, or visionary experiences (involving internal and external sensations), and commonly interpreted as experiences of union with the divine, revelation, or enlightenment.

According to Michael Winkelman (1994:23), consciousness is an interpretive system that has adaptive value from the point of view of natural selection, and "a property associated with biological systems which manifest purposeful and intentional behaviors," but it should not be conflated with ego or self-reflection, which would contradict findings from contemplative traditions, such as Buddhist and Asian philosophical and religious systems. A systemic function of natural organisms, consciousness includes awareness and interpretation of both internal and external stimuli, including one's own thoughts and sensory information, enabling living beings to interact with their environment and maintain homeostasis through self-regulation, to respond, plan, and pursue goals; it involves symbolic capacities, such as represented in language and learning, as well as communal and cultural aspects, like conscience, empathy, and meaning-making (Winkelman 1994:24). There are numerous distinct states of consciousness, including meditation, drowsiness, sleep, dreaming, daydreaming, mania, stupor, or coma. Non-ordinary states have come to be labeled as "altered states of consciousness" (ASCs). While they differ from ordinary awareness, they are not abnormal in a biological or cultural sense, because they constitute fundamental and influential features of animal minds, particularly humanity.

Michael Winkelman and Daniel Moerman have written prolifically on the subject of shamanic experiences associated with altered states of consciousness, the evolutionary, biological, and cultural (thus biocultural) underpinnings and diversity, including therapeutic uses, and recently they have taken their analysis into the realm of neuroscientific theorizing. Buddhist scriptures identify as many as "89 distinct types of consciousness, determined by combinations from 52 elements of consciousness," including seven universal elements: attention, contact, perception, feeling, concentration, will, and psychic energy (Laughlin et al., cited in Winkelman 1994:24). Such "mature contemplative traditions" offer a tremendous range of possibilities of awareness other than the egoic self and rational processing, often requiring that such functions need to be temporarily suspended for other, more advance states, to become achievable.

In Winkelman's recent theoretical work he has branded the term *neurophenomenology* to describe his approach to ASCs, which includes (1) personal phenomenal experience and (2) knowledge of brain structures and functions (Winkelman 2000:xiv). He argues for a broad and complex understanding of consciousness as a system that blends both biological and learned symbolic capacities while emphasizing the importance of the communal dimension hinted at in the form "conscience," and the centrality of social relationships and "social intelligence" in the emergence of the self in relation to "other" and the *reflexive awareness* of the self (Winkelman 2000:11–22). Winkelman writes: "Shamanistic entities and processes, particularly animism, the guardian spirit complex, and possession, provide mechanisms and symbolic systems within which the self develops in interactional symbolic relationships with others" (2000:22). Shamanism offers protection through practices that maintain and integrate the symbolic self and culture in the face of suffering, contradictions, and social crises. In his view, neurophenomenology does not attempt to reduce experience to either matter or mind but recognizes that reality is transcendent and cannot be apprehended "directly," being mediated by senses and cognitive structures, patterns imposed on the world to make sense of it and remember.

The neurophenomenological approach attempts to overcome the dualistic tradition that has so long dominated Western thinking and biomedicine by recognizing that both biological and symbolic processes are involved in the production of human experience and knowledge (Winkelman 2000:24). The effect of mental over physical realms has been amply documented via studies of stress, *placebo* and *nocebo* effect (such as hex death), and psychoneuroimmunology, while experiments in cognitive psychology have shown that mental processes (such as interpretations of meaning) and bodily states are involved in "reciprocal causation" and "downward causation" (Winkelman 2000:26). Drawing on MacLean's model of the "triune" brain, Winkelman affirms that:

> The modern brain operates through the interconnection of the instinctual responses of the reptilian brain, the autonomic emotional states of the paleomammalian brain, and the cognitive processes of the neomammanlian brain, integrating features of these three functional systems. These relationships are mediated physiologically and symbolically, with many effects on consciousness and health. Interactions among the levels of the brain are primarily based not on verbal language, but on other forms of mentation, social representation, and information processing, which utilize social, affective, and symbolic information to mediate, evoke, and channel physiological processes. (2000:33)

These processes are commonly outside the immediate reach of linguistic communication, based in the left hemisphere, yet they provide for significant experiences and aspects of personality and sociality, being involved in a "complex information and intrapsychic communication system that subserves human experience and action," describable as "subsymbolic" and nonverbal (Winkelman 2000:34).

Author of *The Soul in the Brain*, neurologist Michael Trimble (2007) recalls a long line of famous figures (charismatic leaders and artists), documented to have had seizure disorders. Hippocrates devoted a lengthy treatise to epilepsy, which he called the sacred disease. In her filigreed account of a Hmong family's struggles with their young daughter's intractable epilepsy, Anne Fadiman (1997) documented that Lia's seizures meant that she may someday be a great shaman, according to Hmong traditions, and that she would bring hope and healing to her community. Using varied examples from the New World Arctic, Old World Nepal, and Central Africa, Edith Turner (2006:102) pointed out that healers' calling experiences often start by "falling" into unplanned "initiations that are bestowed by spirit agencies," painful or frightening episodes that psychiatrists would describe as dissociation or mental disturbance, often associated with vivid hallucinations. In the case of Arctic Inuit, visions accompanied by a "four-day crazy period" are a common theme in the stories of shamans. Recovery from severe illness or near-death experience comes with the expectation that one become a healer, and the refusal to follow this transformative call can bring the initiate misfortune or even death. Turner remarked:

> In our illnesses and breaks from normalcy, there then opens a space for something spiritual to "come through" to us. This is not a matter of mere belief, however; those who have had their lives transformed in this way insist that they know from experience what is spiritual, owing to the work of a spirit or divine being who has taken the initiative. (2006:101)

The calling is not only a mental reorientation and transformation but an intensely physical experience. Bhirendra of Nepal shook violently, becoming overtaken by the spirit of his grandfather: refusing to become a healer would have made him mad and endangered his life (Turner 2006:107), whereas Muchona, a Ndembu man belonging to a Zambian forest community, describes "being pricked by needles" and tormented, before "a great power came upon" him and he sensed a "fierce pricking" in his fingers, which returns every time he practices divination and guides him to a diagnosis (Turner 2006:111).

Marjorie Mandelstam Balzer (2006:78) describes the revival of shamanic healing in the "Russian Far East" following the collapse of Soviet communism: "shamanic healing has become a crucial part of larger processes of cultural recovery"; during a time of significant hardship and uncertainty, "accounts of miracle cures have begun to supplant the litanies of loss." Balzer describes the shamanic journey of a woman surgeon who ends up giving up the medical profession to become a shaman. Her story began in childhood with visions and frightful dreams, later followed by a severe illness with headaches, hives, and vomiting. Feeling inspired to put on the cloak bequeathed to her by her father, she became tranquil and was healed. The woman then continued using the cloak for healing and experiencing encounters with animal spirit guides, while practicing mainstream medicine. Three years later, she became sick again in the operating room, after performing brain surgery, and woke up with strange marks on her cheeks in a hospital bed. At that time, the healer discovered she had a "new gift, the ability to see through a person into their illnesses" (Balzer 2006:83). She continued healing people with modern medicine (for traumas and hunting accidents) as well as shamanic séances. Upon retirement from her position as head doctor of her region, she continued helping people out of her home, handling emergencies and "curing nervous system disorders and alcoholism. Nikolai, a patient with cancer and several others say they have seen a man standing behind her while she chants, as she evokes the beauty of the northern mountains" (Balzer 2006:84).

Since the 1980s shamanic healing has become increasingly popular in Hungary, notes Imre Lázár (2006:47), where "cultic counter-culture and an experimental medical sub-culture" have merged forces, blending with Jungian depth psychology to provide assistance for youth and adults suffering from schizophrenia, depression, addictions, and other mental disorders. Resistance on religious grounds is not uncommon, but Lázár (2006:47) points out that the emphasis is on technique and method, in a pragmatic sense, the use of repetitive sound (drums, rattles, song, and dance) to bring about a journey in which the participants navigate non-ordinary realms of reality for a short time (twenty minutes), being instructed to return at the call of the drum; upon return, they communicate and reflect on their journey through visual artwork and verbal sharing of experiences. In this context, it is not only the shaman who journeys on behalf of the patient, but the patient himself or herself. In the tradition of participatory and phenomenological anthropology, Lázár (2005:49) reports on his own experience with postural induction of trance states, based on Felicitas Goodman's (1990) "psychological archaeology." Working with Neolithic figures, Goodman identified more than thirty distinct postures that, accompanied by breathing and drumming, produce altered states of consciousness with particular sensations and visions. Lázár found through his own experimental brain mapping studies that the electrophysiology of these varied states had the same features as that of hypnosis and progressive relaxation (2005:49). Many participants in postural trance workshops were seeking to use the trance states as "hermeneutic devices" to understand past or distant spiritualities, but a neo-shamanic community emerged out of the process. In 1997 and 1998, postural trance was combined with ear acupuncture to aid in the treatment of drug addictions. Some members of these workshops and therapy groups went on to found a new spiritual movement, incorporating reiki into their practice (Lázár 2005:50).

While anthropologists have argued for over a century that an observer needs to temporarily suspend judgment to participate in a culture and understand practices in context, Lázár's work is a vivid illustration of the recent development in anthropological research. This newer approach goes beyond classic participant-observation or interpretive textual reading of cultural practices of "others" to embrace deeper forms of participatory, empathetic, and phenomenological involvement with alternative modes of experience, thought, and explanation (Barbara Tedlock, Bonnie Glass-Coffin, and Susan Greenwood). Advocates of phenomenological approaches have aptly pointed out how disingenuous (and imperialistic) it can be to verbally honor and acknowledge the value of someone else's worldview while at the same time dismissing their most significant or formative life experiences, spiritual notions, and epistemologies as mere constructions of reality or naïve illusions. Through participation and initiation into practices of shamanism, magic, sorcery, and even spirit possession rituals, anthropologists have been able to create "embodied" and richly sensual accounts, more truthfully and authentically conveying the voices and worldviews of their informants.

In many cultures, the occurrence of illness and misfortune is attributed to the actions of witches and sorcerers. Anthropologically defined, witches have a supernatural ability to cause harm, sometimes without knowing, and they usually do so for selfish reasons. They may leave their bodies, roam at night, steal others' souls, or turn into animals, causing sickness. Sorcerers use various ritual implements to cause harm to others, for gaining rewards, power, or revenge. Both types of characters are feared and mistrusted. This kind of witch described here is not the same cultural entity as the practitioner of "white magic," used to describe (or self-describe) the nature-centered religion of certain groups and individuals such as neopagans (for example, Wiccans) who are reviving religious traditions associated with the Druids and the Celts, celebrate the regenerative powers of nature, the divine as feminine, and the Earth as archetypal Mother Goddess. In addition, other modern practitioners of "white magic" seek to cultivate the divine within, while embracing an animistic and eco-friendly perspective, which comprises an eclectic blend of Eastern, Christian, and Jewish mysticism and Native American traditions. The practitioners of this latter form of magic tend to emphasize the role of magic and ritual for healing and practice spirituality for self-improvement and self-fulfillment, often individually, identifying (at least partially) with the New Age movement.

Catherine Albanese suggested that "that the discourse and related action promoted by the New Age have emerged as a new healing religion," noting that "the issue of light—at once mystically unifying and scientifically discrete—has captured the mind and imagination of the New Age," making it possible to speak about "the coalescence of the New Age from linked 'light' centers" (1992:75). At the same time, Robert Ellwood (1992:59) argued that "the New Age is a contemporary manifestation of western alternative spirituality going back to at least the Greco-Roman world." The symbolism of light or the millenarian quality of the New Age have quasi-indigenous antecedents in Christian mysticism and Christian (as well as communist) millenarianism, while drawing on symbols and metaphors that exert global appeal. Gehardus Oosthuizen (1992:260) observed that a new wave of South Africa's Hindu academics and professionals were re-connecting with their Hindu roots as a result of the interest generated by Hinduism in the West, particularly in the context of the New Age Movement. Rosalind Hackett (1992:229) wrote that, since independence, Nigeria "has become a veritable marketplace of religions." Hackett pointed to a number of possible "ancestral links" between New Age "spiritual science movements" and indigenous traditions: the notion of spiritual potential, the connection between divination and astrology, the link between ancestral cults and reincarnation, the similarity between spirit possession and channeling, the spiritual use of New Age music, and "the notion that one may become divine"—apotheosis being "an integral feature of Yoruba religion, for example" (1992:225–7).

Hypnosis, Spirit(s), and Healing

States of altered consciousness were an important feature of temple healing and oracular divination in classical India, Greece, and Rome. Named after the Greek word *hypno*, which means sleep, hypnosis gained popularity in the Western world at the turn of the eighteenth century as a result of the work of Franz Anton Mesmer in France (thus the verb *to mesmerize*) and continuing with colleagues in France and England. Mesmer attributed the "animal magnetism" to a cosmic vital fluid made of fire, air, and spirit. Sometimes his method involved laying of hands, which is associated with perception of heat, trembling, or seizures. The popularity of this practice was denounced and ridiculed. Some people argued that it was improper and would lead to sexual misdeeds. The Scottish surgeon James Braid, influenced by accounts of yoga and other "oriental practices" that produced changes in consciousness without the intervention of a therapist, developed the concept and coined the term hypnotism in the middle of the nineteenth century, recognizing that it was not the same as sleep. The popular method was successful in providing pain relief during surgery and childbirth. In the 1950s, hypnosis gained increased acceptance by medical and governmental institutions, including the approval of the pope (Gauld 1992).

In his book *Spirits with Scalpels*, Sidney Greenfield (2008) vividly describes witnessing shocking spirit surgeries by Brazilian healers who were able to make deep cuts with a nonsterile knife into their patients' bodies without the slightest reaction of pain from the subject of these procedures, and without subsequent infection. He notes that hypnosis has a solid track record (evidenced in research studies over the past decade) of its helpfulness with ailments ranging from headaches, irritable bowel, anxiety, and depression (Greenfield 2008:183). Patients who are prone to fantasy and forgetfulness, and hold positive expectancies, tend to do best with hypnotherapies. Greenfield points out that the practice of surgery (both the medical and the spiritist version) follows the model of theater, with healer at the center. He also describes powerful experiences and cures during popular Catholic pilgrimages, charismatic Pentecostal rituals, and African-derived Candomblé and Umbanda. Many of the participants he describes are educated people who use modern medicine along with faith healing, "shopping around" among the various groups and ritual therapies in search of healing efficacy. The healing work that takes place in these religious rituals is analogous to hypnotic suggestion, Greenfield argues, as information becomes "transduced" to the molecular level, rather than simply operating on the mind.

Greenfield echoes the pioneering Michael Winkelman (2000) and Felicitas Goodman (1988), observing that the modern Western model of "normal" or ordinary mental states inherently categorizes "trance" experiences and participants who would spontaneously achieve ASCs through ritual as somehow abnormal, or insane, although it has been documented since the 1970s that nearly 90 percent of small-scale societies exhibit religious trance behaviors. Public and religious rituals commonly induce various altered states of consciousness, stimulating parts of the cerebral cortex while inhibiting the emotional centers. Greenfield draws on the work of Ernest Rossi (2002) to argue for the cyclical nature of human consciousness, which in sleep or wakefulness follows a 90- to 120-minute rhythm, which also represents the time it takes for gene expression or protein synthesis cycle to complete one ultradian cycle

Altered States of Consciousness

of healing. This was apparently familiar to early therapists and put into practice by Milton Erickson. Greenfield (2008:187–90) proposes an explanation of the healing experiences he witnessed on the basis of Rossi's research on the molecular basis of mind/body healing: a type of communication links the cellular or genomic level to behaviors and psychosocial cues. In his view, "information at the cultural level, held as beliefs" involving spirits, saints, or the Holy Spirit is transduced to physiological processes (turning on specific genes) during religious rituals that exceed ninety minutes, in the same way that a hypnotherapist's suggestions are transduced.

The value of hope and trust in healing has long been well established cross-culturally. In *Treating Depression with Hypnosis*, psychotherapist Michael Yapko (2001:44) suggests that "ambiguity may well be the most powerful and pervasive risk factor for depression out of all known risk factors," specifically referring to a "lack of clear meaning associated with one's various life experiences." Whether self-reinforced or culturally reinforced, interpretations of life events have profound consequences in terms of mood, behavior, and prognosis. Hurtful ideas and beliefs (many without factual support) contribute greatly to depression (Yapko 2001:43–4). The success of cognitive, behavioral, and interpersonal therapies results from enabling the sufferer to explore alternative views, explanations, and narratives, with healing effects. Sufferers learn to distinguish more effectively between subjective "projections" and actual "facts." Yapko points out that expectancy has a crucial role to play in the etiology, course, and treatment of depression, hopelessness remaining a leading causative factor and a major obstacle for recovery (2001:61). His focus is to build hopefulness and positive expectancy through hypnotic induction. In accordance to the Western professional standard, a therapist must refrain from projecting his or her views and interpretations on the patient (offering solutions and advice), but must support the patient to elicit more effective coping strategies and explanatory narratives of their own. At the same time, Yapko acknowledges that causes and cures for depression are not merely in the mind: there are many contributing factors, including psychological, biological, and social. A holistic view of depression goes beyond a narrow, generic, and mechanistic view of chemical deficiency or imbalance in the brain and the use of standard protocols or recipes judged appropriate and instead acknowledges the importance of personal and sociocultural factors, including poverty, unemployment, illness, conflict, painful memories, or social isolation.

Locating the basis for depression in the mental/conceptual sphere, Yapko (2001:46) writes that "the essence of depression is that people think things and then mistake their thoughts, beliefs and perceptions for 'truth.'" Thus, a cognitive deficiency is suggested and taking stock of one's intra-psychic narratives is recommended. Yapko (2001) sees the role for hypnosis in helping sufferers reorient toward hope and activity, while controlling negative ruminations. Shifting in the direction of goal-oriented behaviors and independent action places responsibility squarely on the sufferer, reproducing the modern Western capitalist view of individual agency. Unlike traditional healers, Western psychotherapists generally avoid giving advice, in anticipation that cognitive forces (such as willpower and reason) enable clients to reorganize and reframe their own problems, leading to improvement or cure. As a secular practitioner of therapeutic hypnosis, Yapko's modernist perspective differs from ritual or symbolic therapies that rely on suggestibility for healing. His view also contrasts with the European Romantic view of melancholy as a state of aesthetic sensitivity, philosophical sophistication, and creative introspection concerning the fragility and ephemeral nature of love and life, or the Romantics' call to languish in its shadows and temptations. This sensuous, artistic valuing of sorrow and solitude as bittersweet inspiration and material for contemplation differs in turn from starker Buddhist and Hindu views of suffering as illusory, a feature of the mesmerizing sensory world of constant change, life, and death, which may be transcended through enlightenment and liberation from the material body and the shackles of desire and loss.

The Orthodox Christian Desert Fathers considered depression to be a variety of demonic influence, thus placing the ultimate responsibility outside the rational self. In his influential work on depression in China, Arthur Kleinman (1986) showed that self and suffering are locally shaped and interpreted experiences, laying the foundations of much subsequent work on *somatization:* the emphasis on physical and physiological complaints and remedies over emotional, mental, or social dimensions, more prominently addressed in the United States. Janice Boddy (1994), Lesley Sharp (1996), and Adeline Masquelier (2001) noted the effectiveness of spirit possession rituals in relieving the suffering and marginalization of African women with personal and social difficulties, including infertility. In the ritual act of embodying spirits, women can challenge patriarchal authority and traditional norms, behaving in ways commonly forbidden in "proper" society, bending gender roles and expectations, and resisting the pressures, demands, and violence they encounter in everyday life. Spirit(s) often demand gifts (jewelry, perfume, food, or clothes) that benefit and comfort afflicted women. In addition, the latter are relieved from bearing full responsibility for difficulties or losses, while gaining a new voice for dissent, irony, or mockery, and a multisensory social forum for confronting and embodying contradictions, passions, frustration, anguish, uncertainty, or grief. Western views of the self as autonomous and impermeable contrast with indigenous views worldwide, while the contingent nature of experiences and boundaries (of selfhood, loss, and marginalization) mirrors the cultural embeddedness of suffering and therapeutic actions.

Suggestibility and hypnosis are closely connected to the powerful and once maligned so-called placebo effect, a remarkable phenomenon that was not taken seriously by Western scholars until fairly recently. The term *placebo* originates from the Latin expression "I shall please," and refers to the power of belief and expectation to induce positive changes. The meanings, uses, and ethics of placebo have become the topic of much excellent academic research spanning a dizzying array of disciplines, from the history of ideas to molecular biochemistry. Like trance and other altered states of consciousness, placebo effects are based on complex sensory and neurological processes universal in nature, which constitute beneficial evolutionary adaptations. Noting the powerful analgesic effects of placebos, Moerman (2002:100) has noted: "Telling stories about our lives, or creating meaning from grief, can affect our bodies, our biology." Some of the hottest new research in academia lies at the confluence of neuroscience and culture, cognition, creativity, music, art, healing, and the study of sensations. Scientists are trying to map physiological processes and neurochemical pathways involved in particular behaviors, mental states, or emotional experiences, and to explore the interplay of biology and environment with the unique cultural forces and contexts in which patients, healers, and practitioners operate. How and why are particular dynamics and effects generated? Recent studies explore possible synergies between hypnosis, placebo, and acupuncture.

It has become widely known in mental health circles that there are significant benefits from hypnosis, psychotherapy, dietary changes and supplements (eating greens or taking omega-3 oils), and behavioral changes (regular exercise, spending more time outdoors, taking up a new hobby, volunteering to help others, or caring for a pet), either used alone or in combination with drug treatment. At the same time, the drive in the medical profession has been toward elucidating and addressing the biochemical aspects of depression. The consumption of antidepressants by people of all ages has increased dramatically in the past two decades. Twenty million Americans have been diagnosed with depression. It is particularly worrisome that children and elderly have been increasingly targeted for drug therapies, many of which have not been sufficiently tested in these age groups. These medications are commonly administered together with other medications, increasing the dangers of interactions and side effects. The long-term effects are not fully understood, but it is known that some children eat and sleep less or have unusual dreams. A black-box warning was added to Prozac and other selective serotonin reuptake inhibitors (SSRIs) when a number of suicides and other acts of violence were associated with consumption of the drug by children and teens. Billions of dollars are being spent annually just on advertising antidepressants, but drug expenditures have actually decreased somewhat since the introduction of generics for some of the major SSRIs. It is a striking trend that from 1991 to 2005, the total number of antidepressant prescriptions covered by U.S. Medicaid rose 380 percent from 6.82 million to 32.72 million, expenditures being just under $2 billion in 2005 (Chen et al. 2008). Five to six times that amount was spent across all payers. Due to rising popularity and a growing body of evidence for the efficacy of acupuncture, yoga, tai chi, light therapy, and mindfulness therapies for the management of stress, depression, anxiety, and enhancing the quality of life, Americans spent about $20 billion out-of-pocket on such alternative therapies in 2007; in addition, about half of that sum was spent on natural products such as herbal medicines; nearly $3 billion was spent on homeopathy (CU School of Medicine 2011).

Current Practice: Rediscovering Hesychasm and the Prayer of the Heart

The contemplative practice known as Hesychasm, literally quietism, or "the way of stillness," has emerged as an influential and distinctive vehicle for the articulation of cultural identities, values, and aspirations of Romanians since the fall of the communist regime. In the words of Timothy Ware, Bishop Kallistos of Diokleia: "The Hesychast is one who devotes himself to the prayer of silence—to prayer that is stripped, so far as possible, of all images, words, and discursive thinking" (1993:64). Formerly associated almost entirely with Eastern Orthodox monasticism, asceticism, and theological scholarship, Hesychasm is undergoing a vibrant revitalization and popularization among Eastern Europeans of Orthodox faith in Romania and elsewhere, and most significantly among younger generations. Like ELTA and Radiant Technique, this is a spiritually informed practice that has been generating a small but steadily growing following since 1989, particularly among the educated youth.

A practitioner and lay teacher of Hesychasm (*Isihasm* in Romanian), writer Vasile Andru is a distinctive figure on the cultural scene of contemporary Romania. He has lectured abundantly on Hesychast practice, asserting its profoundly transformative value and promoting its application outside traditional monastic contexts. For years following the removal of communism in 1989, Andru was consistently filling the Sala Dalles auditorium in downtown Bucharest with hundreds of participants who paid a small entrance fee to attend his conferences. He referred to the group as *Cercul de Practică Isihastă* (The Circle of Hesychast Practice). His loyal and enthusiastic audiences commonly span more than six decades in age and a diversity of educational backgrounds.

Andru's own spiritual and cross-cultural explorations have taken him on several journeys to India, the Himalayas, and other parts of Southeast Asia, as well as to Eastern Orthodoxy's Sacred Mount Athos. His ability to connect Indian or yogic techniques of breathing and contemplation with the Orthodox Hesychast tradition enhances the expansive, visionary qualities of his conferences and broadens the popular appeal of his public talks. Aimed at a general audience with cursory knowledge of Orthodoxy, Andru's lectures present the Hesychast practice of contemplation and prayer as a practical method for experiencing divinity and a path for bettering the self and the social environment. Illumination, awakening, and the realization of divine presence are brought about through the practice of Hesychasm both inside and outside of the monastic context, according to Andru. In his view, consistent practice of Hesychast prayer leads not only to perfect mental clarity but also to better health and longer life. Additionally, the evolution of individuals to a higher consciousness benefits everyone in their proximity. "It is sufficient for one enlightened being to be in a space to redeem the entire space," Andru asserts. His statement reflects a radically different conception of redemption and enlightenment compared to Protestant or capitalist notions of individualized action or self-autonomy. In this Orthodox-inspired view, persons are not isolated from others or apart from the space they inhabit. Their spiritual destinies are woven into this space, able to transform it and to alter others' permeable identities by transforming themselves.

Andru refers to the practice of repeated utterance of the prayer of the heart as *oratio mentis*, describing it as an individual, personal, mysterious exercise. He chooses to translate the Latin expression as "prayer of the mind in the heart." The use of Latin terminology appears as a discreet attempt to further legitimize it by invoking the authority of the high scholarship that Latin connotes, while the emphasis on "in the heart" secures the connection with the body, which is distinctive of the Eastern Orthodox tradition from which the practice originates. Andru broadens the relevance and appeal of Hesychasm as a transformative practice by addressing its connections and similarities to Indian techniques of meditation and the body (Yoga in particular). In doing so, he strengthens the authority of this practice by putting it in a global framework and frees this technique of the self from its formerly exclusive monastic context.

John T. Chirban (1991:4) wrote that the separation between physical healing and spiritual healing of a human being began with Hippocrates and became increasingly accentuated, contrasting with the Orthodox perspective of the Desert Fathers, which was holistic. Chirban (1991:5) remarked that "a renaissance for the appreciation of the whole person is currently in progress," with medical schools beginning to recognize the role of emotions, meditation, and the methods of psychology on the causes and cures of ailments and their impact on immune system functioning. He comments on the popular work of Herbert Benson (a Harvard cardiologist) on the value of the "relaxation response" for preventative medicine, pointing to Benson's recognition that "prayer was prescribed in early Christian times (codified at Mount Athos in the fourteenth century)." Chirban observed: *Prayer*

> A Christian was to pray two times daily, sitting quietly, pay attention to breathing, and say silently, "Lord Jesus Christ, have mercy upon me, a sinner." In addition to its spiritual value, this method of prayer meets the criteria for effecting the relaxation response, which controls hypertension and the development of other diseases. When modern man may pay as much as $500 on a course to learn the relaxation response, its physiological benefits can be a natural by-product of following this basic tenet of Christianity. (1991:5–6)

Encouraged by emergence of psychoneuroimmunology, neuropsychology, and psychopharmacology twenty years ago, Chirban (1991:8) hopefully suggested that "a quiet evolution" was under way in health and healing, replacing a mechanistic, compartmentalized, biochemical view of the person with a more "holistic," multidimensional, integrative approach. That quiet revolution has grown into a tide.

The link between religion and healing runs very deep in the world of Ortho-dox Christianity. Christ himself was a healer, and participation in acts of healing is seen as aligning one's life with Christ (Chirban 1991:3). In early Christianity and the Byzantine empire, people commonly sought healing through contact with men and women who were considered holy. Healing was also reported through praying, touching the relics or the coffin of a saint, anointing, holy water, spending the night in a church ("incubation"), as well as burning small cloth fragments from a saint's clothing and breathing in the scent (Chirban 1991:9).

A view of healing based in the Orthodox tradition is intricately entwined with the Orthodox understanding of personhood, which is, in turn, based on Eastern Chris-tian understandings of the trinitarian nature of the one God. The view of the human person as "an icon of God, a finite expression of God's infinite self expression . . . is the foundation, the polestar, of all Orthodox Christian anthropology," writes Kallis-tos Ware (1996:2). The other key aspect of Orthodox personhood is its "horizontal" orientation: "to be human is to be in relationship with our fellow humans," notes Ware (1996:3); "the God in whose image we are made is God the Holy Trinity, and so the divine icon within each of us is a Trinitarian icon," this God is "not a simple monad, not one person loving himself alone, but three persons—Father, Son, and Holy Spirit—loving one another in reciprocal relationship." Ware explains the high-est goal of human life and experience thus:

> We are called to reproduce on earth the *perichoresis* (interchange of mutual love) that unites the three members of the Holy Trinity in heaven. The unity of the Trinity, needless to say, is a unique unity, and human persons can never be one with the same degree of closeness and reciprocal indwelling as prevails among the three divine persons. But, after full allowance has been made for the differentiation of the divine and the human, it can still be claimed that there is an analogy between the two levels: "Even as you, Father, are in me and I am in you, may they also be one in us" (John 17:21). (1996:4)

Since God is relational, one cannot speak of the divine being without the concept of communion. Similarly, no human being can fulfill their personhood apart from others. From an Orthodox perspective, Descartes's *cogito, ergo sum* contains only a fragment of the truth of human experience, affirms Ware (1996:4), observing that other essential dimensions of personhood can be stated as *amo, ergo sum* (I love, therefore I am) and *amor, ergo sum* (I am loved, therefore I am). He goes on to quote Fr. Dumitru Staniloae (1903–1993), a Romanian theologian considered to one of the most enlightened theological minds of our century: "Insofar as I am not loved, I am incomprehensible to myself" (Ware 1996:4).

The interpersonal nature of humanness is made more visible in the Greek lan-guage, where *atomon* designates the individual as a unit and connotes separation, whereas *prosopon* denotes communion (Ware 1996:4). St. Makarios the Egyptian is said to have asked a pagan priest's skull what it was like in hell, to be told that it is

to act in eternal ways can be healing

a place where people are fixed back to back rather than face to face (Ware 1996:5, referring to the sayings of the Desert Fathers, *Apophthegmata Patrum*). Ware further suggests that more than being simply in the image of God, human beings have the potential to be in God's likeness, meaning that they have inherent and inexhaustible potentialities for growth, transformation, and ultimately *theosis* (Ware 1996:6–7).

Self-awareness and freedom are the gifts of divine likeness that allow the human being to participate in creation truly as an offerer and as a maker of his or her own unique destiny (Ware 1996:8–10). It is essential to recall here once again that for the Orthodox person, as for the Desert Fathers, the body constitutes the fundamental grounds and primary instrument for salvation, self-fashioning, and ultimately deification. The physical body is involved in all of the sacraments, and it is the site of actualization of the highest human potentials for freedom, a freedom that is achieved through the "care of the self," in Foucault's (1988, 1997 [1984]) famous words, and a freedom that requires a commitment to relationships with both the divine and human others. The model of Christ and his fully human yet fully divine nature represents the basis for human *theosis*, an act of grace that one can prepare for through practices of discipline, asceticism, and self-cultivation. Indeed, as the resurgence in religious participation and the interest in Hesychasm exemplify, traditional modes of engagement with the world and human others are being made more current than ever as people search for freedom and personal fulfillment in Eastern Europe and the Balkans.

Rising Trend: Healing Addictions with ASCs and Hallucinogens

Anthropologists have long documented the cross-cultural ritual use of hallucinogens (psychoactive or vision-inducing substances, sometimes referred to as psychedelics), which included peyote and San Pedro's cacti, psilocybin-containing mushrooms, various parts of the Ayahuasca vine, tobacco, coca, and others. The expansive work *Plants of the Gods* by Schultes, Hofmann, and Rätsch (2001), and the cross-cultural review by Dobkin De Rios (1984), offer ample and elaborate accounts of plant-based hallucinogens commonly involving therapeutic uses. For over two decades, Winkelman has successfully argued that the practice of ASCs by magico-religious healers was an ecological adaptation of hunter-gatherers that developed as a result of the universal biophysiological properties and capacities of the human brain, ASC-based healing being continued in agricultural and large-scale societies by other types of healers and possession-trance mediums. His review article on the therapeutic uses of hallucinogens drew further attention to commonalities across cultures in terms of neurobiology and behavior under the effects of these substances, the biological pathways of which had not yet been elucidated, noting the relevance of individual and environmental factors such as "set" (individual features and expectations) and "setting" (physical and social aspects), which refer to the fact that context and the shamanistic healer shaped the course and meaning of these experiences for the participant (Winkelman 1991).

There are several classes of compounds that are similar or equivalent in their effects, while varying in potency. One such grouping comprises LSD, psilocybin mushrooms, and mescaline. Active ingredients are similar to existing neurotransmitters in the human body. When these substances have been used in psychotherapy, the therapist or shaman has acted as a guide to help the patient integrate the experiences within the larger life context, meeting with the patient (and sometimes with the family as well) before and after the experience, using ritual, mythical, and symbolic elements to change the patient's awareness of self (it temporarily dissolves) and break up habitual experiences of the world; patients become more suggestible (Winkelman 1991:16). Hallucinogens initiate "high voltage synchronous activity in the hippocampus," which is involved in memory and learning, and stimulate the limbic system, which controls the autonomic nervous system and human physiology: an effect that provides a basis for the healing and curing of diverse illnesses through ASCs (Winkelman 1991:17). Hallucinogens also have sensory effects, emotional effects, behavioral effects, and cognitive effects, which contribute to increased coherence and integration of brain discharges and the two hemispheres as well as the harmonization of feelings and thoughts (Winkelman 1991:17–18).

More recently, Winkelman has produced a unique body of ample and influential data and analyses of the neurobiology and has advocated for therapeutic value of psychoactive substances, which had long been considered unequivocally harmful by Western policy makers. Pointing to their universality and biological basis, he has been instrumental in changing perceptions of ASCs from primitive and delusional behaviors to key elements in the evolution of human integrative and symbolic capacities. Winkelman (2001a) proposed coining a new, less stigmatizing term for these substances, to indicate their capability to influence serotonergic neurotransmission and the fact that:

> Effects upon neural, sensory, emotional, and cognitive processes stimulate integrative information processing, justifying a new term—"psychointegrators." Psychointegrators disinhibit sensory and emotional processes. They stimulate systemic integration of brain information-processing functions, enhancing integration of limbic system self and emotional dynamics with neocortical processes.

Based on ethnographic and scientific evidence of healing from traditional settings, Alcoholics Anonymous, shamanic drumming workshops, and clinical studies of meditation, Winkelman (2001b) argues that ASCs can be effective in treating addictions due to their ability to "induce the relaxation response, enhance theta-wave production, and stimulate endogenous opioid and serotonergic mechanisms and their mood elevating effects." He has developed a shamanic drumming approach to treating addictions.

Faith Healing and Pilgrimage

Ritual healing and religious pilgrimage are classical anthropological subjects, having attracted intense observation and analysis by many anthropological scholars and scholars of religion. They represent deeply transformative experiences, richly cloaked and embedded in the symbols, sensations, and emotions of a particular cultural context, situated in space and time. A lead analyst of the social functions of religion, Émile Durkheim (1965 [1915]) described a *collective conscience* that emerges in the process of religious ritual and infuses the community with power and solidarity. In his view, such religious practices and experiences manifested traditional networks and structures of the society, thus reinforcing the group's sacred stories, values, and norms. Recent studies on health and social involvement show that, along with the maintenance and propagation of societal and cultural traditions, participation in group rituals and religious communities also contributes to the preservation of the individual by reducing mortality. The health and longevity benefits of social involvement have been documented in scientific studies, revealing that both quality and quantity of one's social relationships are linked to mental health, morbidity, and mortality with a recent review suggesting as much as "a 50% increased likelihood of survival for participants with stronger social relationships," the impact of relationships on mortality risk being "comparable with well-established risk factors for mortality" (Holt-Lunstad et al. 2010).

Historian of religions Mircea Eliade (1991 [1954]) noted that ritual offers humans the opportunity to renew themselves and the world around them by uniting with the divine through ritual action. Like Durkheim, Eliade argued that sacred time and sacred space are qualitatively different from their profane counterparts. As sacred spaces commemorate creation, they sit at the very center of the universe, being ontologically "more real" for participants than profane spaces. Ritual activities create a rift in time, making manifest the primordial, mythical, or liturgical time, allowing religious persons and their community to experience deep renewal through the manifestation and union with the sacred. Anthropologist Claire Farrer (2011 [1994]) vividly described the enactment of "mythical time" among the Mescalero Apache people of New Mexico during the four-day, four-night puberty ceremony that marks their taking leave of childhood to become Apache women. Her work is a classic illustration of a puberty ritual reflecting the classic stages of rites of passage that frame a profound change of identity and status.

The ritual is timed by the setting and rising of the sun and involves the building and taking down of a giant tepee, supported by four poles, representative of the four cardinal directions (a sacred number in most native North American cultures). During the peak of the transition stage, elaborately costumed, faces dusted with pollen, a symbol of fertility and the power of the sun, deeply exhausted from the physical and emotional trials of days of dancing, the girls become manifestations of White Painted Woman. She is said to have journeyed in as a young woman, from the east, then south into adulthood, then west as she matured, and north as she withered into old age, to come back youthful again the next morning, from the east (Farrer 2011 [1994]:42). In ritual, the young women embody this culture hero of the Apache, who brought them their knowledge of health and healing and other valuable skills. As incarnations of White Painted Woman, also called White Changing Woman, they are able to bestow blessings on those gathered to honor them through this life-changing journey of womanhood. Thus, healing is integral to this communal experience. As hundreds of people, family, and friends, gather to enact this sacred ritual for their young women, the Apache community (as Durkheim observed) strengthens, venerates, and perpetuates itself into the future.

Beyond being a simple act of social reproduction, however, the girls' puberty ritual acts as a healing journey on multiple levels: personal, social, ecological, and cosmic. It needs to be remembered that for more than a century, these traditions were banned by the U.S. government as primitive, pagan, and forbidden, because they conflicted with Judeo-Christian views of puberty and menstruation as something shameful, to be hidden, rather than publicly commemorated. In formally celebrating the women's centrality to their matrilineal culture and ensuring the continuity of their cultural traditions, the Apache people also celebrate their own healing and survival in the twenty-first century, their freedom to embrace and continue performing ancient rites, stories, and cultural traditions. By making manifest their religious traditions, the participants open a direct connection to the original time of creation, when White Painted Woman first arrived, while also reaching out far beyond the present moment into the distant world of future generations.

In his influential work on ritual and pilgrimage, Victor Turner described the ritual pilgrim's journey as a breach in space and time, when the established social order becomes temporarily suspended, thus a time of anti-structure, charged with the possibility of unexpected insights and creative potential for profound change, personal or communal. Thus, religion and ritual are not merely a way to preserve the social order but can be opportunities to suspend or challenge the social order for the time of the ritual, as in the case with carnival-time excesses and debauchery. His analysis described the transitional phase of rites of passage as "betwixt and between," neither here nor there, riddled with ambiguity, situated in the margins of "regular" social experience. From the Latin word *limen* (threshold), Turner further developed the characteristics of *liminality* pertaining to van Gennep's transition phase: a socially ambiguous state, sometimes incorporating hardships or tests into the transformation process.

Turner argued for the potential of ritual to rejuvenate self and society rather than simply uphold or reproduce tradition. He pointed to pilgrimage as a ritual event characterized by an extended period of liminality during which social distinctions tend to fall by the wayside. Participants' destinies and identities temporarily merge to form a ritual gathering he called *communitas*, characterized by uniformity of status and sometimes appearance among participants, which may engender modifications in perceptions and consciousness, allowing or creating new possibilities of transformation, healing, and unexpected change. In nonmedical health and healing, pilgrimages have played a most significant role, cross-culturally. One of the most well-known pilgrimages is the *hajj,* which is required of every devout Muslim at least once in his or her lifetime. The hajj reproduces the journey of Mohammed to Mecca, bringing together people from all imaginable backgrounds and many different countries. In India, several great pilgrimages take place, the largest being the Great Kumbh Mela at Allahabad, which attracts up to many tens of millions of Hindus every twelve years. There are Buddhist pilgrimage sites throughout Asia, including the Eight Great Places in India and Nepal (Scott 2010:xxvii). To this day, pilgrimages to healing sites such as Lourdes in the French Pyrenees continue to attract many millions of people annually.

In his recent book *Miracle Cures: Saints, Pilgrimage and the Healing Powers of Belief,* Robert Scott (2010) delves into a rich historical account of healing miracles ascribed to medieval European saints and argues for the reality of beneficial effects derived from saints and pilgrimages across many centuries, which are abundantly documented. In the small agricultural villages of old Europe, he notes, there were ample reasons for illness, from lack of water purification to malnutrition, accidents, and plagues. Bread provided most of the caloric intake and because economies were local, winters were marked by the absence of fresh foods and necessary vitamins. Nevertheless, illness was commonly attributed to sin rather than naturalistic factors and those with signs of sickness were stigmatized (Scott 2010:70–1). Medieval doctors often used harsh methods for eradicating the culprit, such as purging, bleeding, or using saltwater soaked bandages on wounds. Living conditions were extremely harsh, with no institutional protection from the violence of daily life, something that communal and religious life helped buffer against (Scott 2010:4).

A saint's being was permeated with a divine force called *virtus,* equally present in even the smallest fragment (such as a strand of hair), which permeated every part of the saint's body and everything the saint touched, including the ground around the tomb, and which prevented the decomposition of their bodies and gave an "odor of sanctity" (Scott 2010:38–9). Interestingly, in some cases, the healing power of a saint tends to wane over time, one common explanation being that saints have a limited number of favors they can bestow, saints-in-waiting being often more effective than older ones (Scott 2010:36). The pilgrimage would involve confession of sins before departure and on the way there, presentation of gifts, tactile contact with the reliquary containing the saint's remains (special openings existed in tombs for inserting body parts) and spending several nights sleeping beside it (Scott 2010:41). Because of the association of sickness and sin, healing restored and even enhanced social standing: the healed would become akin to celebrities in a sacred drama, while dying people, who in their own villages would have been utterly marginalized (as the dying are in our society, oftentimes), would take center stage (Scott 2010: 72, 92). Thus pilgrimage helps to remake suffering into a meaningful narrative, as shown in Suzanne Kaufman's (2005) account of Lourdes, who noted that persons healed (mostly women) became enabled to reformulate their suffering and distress in cosmic and more accepting terms as a result of making the journey of the pilgrimage.

Scott (2010:75) credits Victor and Edith Turner (1978) for suggesting that the timing of a pilgrimage may have also reflected the need to escape a stressful social context, while adding that it may have provided a chance to get away from other discomforts, such as an oppressive marriage. Even while liberating, escape from one's everyday environment was likely to have been disorienting and the trip itself arduous, with miles or tens of miles to walk each day and the need to ask for charity or shelter along the way (Scott 2010:75–80). This transitional and ambiguous state, Scott (2010:80) observes, created a sense of intimacy with the saints and fostered supportive bonds among pilgrims who kept one another company. In the case of Lourdes, dramatic stories of faith healing amount to 6,500 reported improvements from 1899 to 1999, 2,500 being recognized as "truly remarkable" and 66 as "miracle cures" (Scott 2010:170). However, I would like to point out that a significant proportion of pilgrimages worldwide do not entail the expectation of miracles, but rather the desire for spiritual transformation, renewal, purification, health improvement, learning, group socialization, or personal development. Scott notes that a drug manufacturer would not get a medicine approved with such a small margin of success, but I would add: even one miracle is still a miracle.

Drawing on literature that attests to the power of placebo analgesia, Scott points out that the mere expectation of relief may have helped to reduce the pain sensations, inflammation, and anxiety experienced by pilgrims while enhancing the production of endorphins and other natural painkillers. At the same time, he suggests the possibility that planning the journey itself can boost one's sense of self-efficacy, thereby strengthening the immune systems. People also draw on their cultural or social environment, including someone else's behavior, to label and interpret what they feel. Kirmayer (1992:329) elegantly observed: "In sickness we confront the inchoate." The act of undergoing a pilgrimage to a healing shrine may seem from a scientific perspective irrational and based upon naïve religious belief in miraculous powers and places. But the persons in the crowds that flow to pilgrimage sites every year are enacting culturally and emotionally rich scenarios of hope, purposefulness, and resilience, thereby transforming themselves from sufferers into protagonists, not victims of their fate.

Ayurveda and Mental Illness

Ayurveda is a South Asian system of medical practices that dates back more than three thousand years. It is still widely practiced in India and other South Asian countries, alongside varied local remedies and Western biomedicine, which is commonly referred to as "allopathy" or "English medicine." Ayurveda is based on ancient medical treatises written in Sanskrit (the sacred language of ancient India and the language of classical medical texts composed between 1000 B.C.E. and 800 C.E.),

which continue to be used and cited by Ayurvedic physicians, whose formal education is comparable in rigor with Western medical school (Halliburton 2009:43–4).
The practice of Ayurveda relies on thousands of substances and combinations of substances (herbs, spices, animal and mineral products), dietary prescriptions, as well as
massage and ritual remedies, to seek improved health and balance, often described in
terms of three bodily humors known as the *dosas* (*vata* or "wind," *pitta* or "bile," and
kapha or "phlegm") and properties such as heat and cold. Ayurvedic medicines are
less processed than Western pharmaceuticals and traditionally they are selected and
mixed for each patient according to their unique condition (Halliburton 2009:47).
Although empirical evidence for the benefits of Ayurvedic therapies spans millennia,
Western-style scientific research is currently being carried out on Ayurvedic therapies
to generate additional validation, including double-blind placebo-controlled trials.
Many Ayurvedic medicines are becoming standardized, produced in factories, and
sold in pharmacies, much like Western allopathic medicines.

Murphy Halliburton's (2009) study of Ayurvedic treatments for mental illness,
vividly captured in his book *Mudpacks and Prozac*, describes the Kerala province
of India as a highly pluralistic environment where many medical treatment options are available, including biomedicine, Ayurveda, and religious healing, which
includes Hindu and Muslim temples and Christian churches. Halliburton points
out that the Ayurvedic perspective and approach emphasizes healing as a gradual
process of building health and well-being (in terms of change, improvement, prosperity) and moving to a "higher level" of health rather than rapid or complete
"cure," which is the stated goal of biomedicine (2009:13). His phenomenological
approach emphasizes the sensory and embodied experience of healing as a lived
experience. His patient informants speak of a pleasant and "cooling" effect that is
associated with Ayurvedic psychiatric treatments, such as *talapodichil,* a medicated
"mudpack" treatment applied to activate a physiologically significant *marma* point
situated in between the forehead and the top of the head; this mudpack treatment
provides an aesthetic experience that is important to patients, and which contrasts
to the generally unpleasant nature of allopathic treatments like "shock" therapy
(Halliburton 2009:20). Ayurveda and religious therapies engage the senses in healing with music, incense, flowers, and beautiful surroundings, whereas allopathic
treatments and hospital settings are characteristically anaesthetic and unaesthetic
(Halliburton 2009:163).

Halliburton (2009:164) draws on his research in Kerala to echo Joseph Alter's
(1999:44) critique of "curing" as an expression of the Western "remedial bias" in
viewing medical practices, which emphasizes the need to remove illness and restore
wellness through oppositional means and devalues approaches that aim for improvement
or transformation (such as palliative care) rather than removal of problems. Deviations
from that dynamic individual profile of *dosas* that constitute a person's well-being
become manifested as discomfort, distress, or illness, which Ayurvedic treatments
can alleviate incrementally (Halliburton 2009:47). Many patients interviewed by
Halliburton turned to Ayurvedic methods after disappointing experiences with

unpleasant side effects of allopathic medicines, including electroconvulsive therapy. Interestingly, Ayurveda's therapeutic methods, which traditionally included more abrasive methods, such as cleansing, have become increasingly gentle over time as practitioners have sought to further distinguish themselves from allopathic doctors. At the same time, with increasing time pressures for people to get back to work or school, the quicker effects of biomedicine present distinct advantages. In Europe and the United States, Ayurvedic treatments are often associated with New Age spirituality and spa therapies, while their perceived holism and reputed gentleness offer a competitive alternative to Western biomedical treatments (Halliburton 2009:48).

Halliburton reflects on the social nature of the self that is said to characterize Southeast Asia and the social nature of healing in Kerala, where patients are usually accompanied and assisted by a relative during medical consultations and treatments. Moreover, Ayurvedic healers commonly adopt a "teacher-student style interaction," telling stories and offering moral advice from their own life experiences, an approach that contrasts with the allopathic and Western approach to psychotherapy and its individualistic model of doctor–patient interaction, in which the psychiatrist or psychologist must refrain from advice, eliciting instead the patient's own insights (Halliburton 2009:56–7). Hindus, Muslims, and Christians made use of the Ayurvedic treatments in Kerala, and all three groups of patients could also be found seeking religious healing at the local mosque Beemapalli, the burial place of a noted female saint, which attracts people of different faiths who seek healing from problems ranging from infertility to mental illness (Halliburton 2009:78). Other treatment modalities available are "tribal medicines," homeopathy and naturopathy, the latter being healing methods more recently imported from the West.

While he acknowledges the distinctive strengths of biomedicine, Halliburton calls into question its instrumental prioritization on a global scale as an enabling handmaiden to stress-laden modern lives and as a key tool in the pursuit of capitalist economic efficiency. Many Indian patients who would rather use Ayurveda for its pleasurable but more time-consuming methods of enhancing health, feel compelled to turn to the speedy solutions of biomedicine in order to continue working or studying with as little interruption as possible in an increasingly competitive and demanding socioeconomic environment.

Enmeshed in daily struggles with the pragmatic realities of post-modern life, such healing journeys represent arenas of change, rather than merely symptoms, reactions, and potentials. The seeker of healing enacts the freedom and opportunity to restore oneself from an array of cultural myths and realities, "indigenous" or "exotic." In the care for the self, cultural and collective destinies can be interrogated and possibly recast. Such quests are exploratory, developmental, and contemplative spaces, theaters if change, where active and creative existential experiments are being performed, blending social critique, scientific argument, local knowledge, and ancient sources of wisdom.

QUESTIONS FOR CLASS DISCUSSION

1. Do you have personal rituals that help you maintain your health holistically? How do you evaluate the benefits? Hypothesize how they originated and how they work for you.
2. Have you ever been on a long journey to a place of special meaning? How is that different from casual or vacation travel? What did you do and feel once you were there?
3. Use a reputable website to find a detailed description of a healing ritual from an indigenous culture, summarize it in your own words, and bring it to class for discussion.

QUESTIONS FOR ESSAY WRITING

1. Describe one of your favorite childhood memories and why it still makes you happy.
2. Write an essay on what hope means to you and how you view its role in severe illness.
3. Choose one of your favorite symbols as your essay topic. Carry out brief background research on its possible meanings and uses in magical rituals. Describe two possible ways in which this symbol can be (or has been) used to direct awareness, provide an interpretation of events, or influence behavior.

SUGGESTED READINGS

Brown, Patricia Leigh (2009), "A Doctor for Disease, A Shaman for the Soul." *The New York Times*, September 19, 2009. Accessed January 21, 2011, at http://www.nytimes.com/2009/09/20/us/20shaman.html.

Harrington, Anne (2008), *The Cure Within: A History of Mind-Body Medicine*. New York: W. W. Norton & Company.

Tedlock, Barbara (2005), *The Woman in the Shaman's Body: Reclaiming the Feminine in Religion and Medicine*. New York: Bantam.

RECOMMENDED FILMS

India: A Second Opinion by T. R. Reid (two 7–8 minute documentary segments; I: "An Uncomfortable Introduction"; II: "Demystifying Ayurveda") from Frontline WORLD; free online at http://www.pbs.org/wgbh/pages/frontline.

The Split Horn (2001) by Taggart Siegel and Jim McSilver: a Hmong Shaman's life and his family's experiences in Laos and America; available from collectiveeye.org, the companion website is http://www.pbs.org/splithorn/.

The Story of the Weeping Camel (2003): beautiful film about a Mongolian healing ritual.

Whale Rider (2002) by Niki Caro; a New Zealand film on native Maori culture and myth.

INTERNET RESOURCES

The Foundation for Shamanic Studies (Michael Harner) http://www.shamanism.org/.

"Reiki and the Catholic Church" segment from PBS program *Religion & Ethics News Weekly*, February 17, 2010 (from minute 3:20 to 11:50); accessed January 21, 2011, at http://video.pbs.org/video/1416128567/.

–4–

Body, Movement, and the Senses

Much of what humans know and believe about the world comes from being born in a sensuous body. Beginning with the instinctual rooting for the mother's breast, babies learn to recognize her smell among all others, anticipating her approach by the closeness and tone of her voice, or stirring at the sight of infant formula in a baby bottle, turning toward familiar voices or intonations of the native language, the neighbor's barking dog, or the television that rarely goes off. The child sways to the rhythms of the mother's body as she works and sings, baby strapped to her back in an Indonesian rice paddy, or rocks to the steady movement of an electric swing in a Texas kitchen, country tunes streaming on the radio, bacon sizzling on the hot stove. Mouth and nostrils take in the fragrant sauces and the spices of daily living: chili peppers, onions, curry paste, miso soup, rice, fast-food fries. Poets, philosophers, biologists, and anthropologists have long embraced the notion that the sensual body is the foremost instrument of knowledge, experience, and survival, the fundamental basis of connection with all caregivers and the primary tool for learning cultural habits and norms of our native social worlds.

Famous old photographs of Franz Boas, the American pioneer of ethnographic exploration and cultural relativism, show him dressed in full Native American costumes, performing the ritual dances that represented totemic animals and myths. The historical particularism approach he advocated called for close examination of a culture's heritage and unique history in order to understand how its distinctive past and its traditions contributed to particular forms of engagement, shaping the culture of the present. His students, Ruth Benedict and Margaret Mead, further explored how cultures differ in the formation of individual personality and behavior, producing creative and influential analyses of other cultural worlds, which have since been amply critiqued for drawing overly broad typologies and generalizations. Colored by a hidden sense of civilized superiority, Malinowski's controversial secret diaries later revealed that he did not always enjoy his fieldwork situation or the people he studied during his extended stay in the Trobriand Islands, but this "father of anthropological fieldwork" firmly established the unparalleled power of extended and continuous immersion for understanding cultural other-worlds. Sensory engagement, acknowledged or not, has played an important part in anthropology from its inception, despite the fact that the goal of unbiased scientific methodology entailed conceptual and analytical distance between natives and the anthropologist.

Confident description, explanation, and taxonomizing of "primitive" thinking and behavior was later overtaken by the interpretive turn, jump-started in anthropology by the influential work of Clifford Geertz (1973). This perspective emphasized the role of the observer in the process of data gathering and analysis, centering on the notion of "culture as text," the importance of thick description, and reflexivity. Until recently, many representatives of the brilliant generation that has followed in Geertz's footsteps emphasized (and arguably overemphasized) that the anthropological acts of observation and analysis of cultural others involve a hermeneutic decoding of bodies and everyday practices as meaning-rich cultural texts, read over the natives' shoulders as well as between the lines, to be filtered through the experience and analytical mind of the ethnographer, and reinvented in the process of ethnographic writing. Post-modernist approaches foreground the act of interpretation, the self-conscious awareness of the ethnographer's biases and participation, and the re-presentation inherent in all ethnographic endeavors. The anthropology of embodiment and the new "sensory turn" in anthropology have challenged the dominance of verbal metaphors and texts over feelings and experiential knowing, showing that preference for vision, writing, and abstract (or disembodied) knowledge reflects Western intellectual heritage, not "reality" or "truth" of other people's worlds.

In his proposal of "embodiment as a paradigm for anthropology" Thomas Csordas (1990:5) stated the need for a perspective which "begins from the methodological postulate that the body is not an *object* to be studied in relation to culture, but is to be considered as the *subject* of culture, or in other words as the existential ground of culture," rather than being simply the cognitive or symbolic ground and instrument of culture. Csordas notes that in 1938 Mauss had distinguished between the "totemistic personage" of tribal societies (incorporating features of the clan's totem: often a bird or animal), the classical persona of antiquity, and the Christian person, the individualistic notion of the person that emerged prior to the Enlightenment. Csordas challenges the separation of perception from practice, arguing that his own approach to embodiment seeks to collapse rather than reproduce entrenched dualisms of subject/object and body/mind, reproduced in Mauss's distinct elaborations of *la notion du personne* (person) and *les techniques du corps* (body techniques).

Csordas positions his brand of experiential methodology in relation to that of philosopher Merleau-Ponty (1962), who located his theory of embodiment in the ontological primacy of perception as preobjective and provided a critique of empiricism. Merleau-Ponty pioneered phenomenology as a descriptive science, arguing that the distinction of subject and object is a result of reflective practice, not prior to it, and that therefore human perception does not begin with objects, but rather it has its "end in objects." Csordas also distinguishes his approach from that of sociologist Pierre Bourdieu (1977), who located his influential analysis of behavioral orientations and cultural patterns in the distinction of structure from practice and the concept of *habitus*, which he borrowed from Mauss's (1973) influential body techniques essay, originally published in the 1930s, which presented the body as object and tool for culture. For Bourdieu, however, *habitus* is more than a mere set of practices; it is a cultural principle that structures practices, most often unconsciously, in accordance to the social world. The *habitus* generates and unifies cultural practices through the body:

> This principle is nothing other than the *socially informed body*, with its tastes and distastes, its compulsions and repulsions, with, in a word, all its *senses*, that is to say, not only the traditional five senses . . . but also the sense of necessity and the sense of duty, the sense of direction and the sense of reality, the sense of balance and the sense of beauty, common sense and the sense of the sacred, tactical sense and the sense of responsibility, business sense and the sense of propriety, the sense of humor and the sense of absurdity, moral sense and the sense of practicality, and so on. (Bourdieu 1977:124)

[handwritten margin notes: a star symbol; "List of Senses"]

Csordas (1990:35) critiqued earlier approaches to perception because (1) it was treated strictly as a cognitive function, rather than in relation to "self, emotion or cultural objects such as supernatural beings"; (2) studies overemphasized visual perception and partitioned the senses without considering synthesis or interplay; and (3) tasks were taken out of social context for abstract or experimental study. He argues that "it is not legitimate to distinguish mind and body" in the act of perception, because our bodies are the ground of experience, not mere objects of it, making the mind/body distinction uncertain (Csordas 1990:36). Just as our bodies only become objects through reflections, Csordas suggests that other people become objectified through reflection as well, but at the experiential level, the other is a part of the self. The apprehension of non-duality and the dissolution of the self is the core principle and goal of contemplative classical Yoga practices and the 4,000-year-old Vedanta tradition, one of the six orthodox systems of Hinduism.

Affirming that "the body is a productive starting point for analyzing culture and self," Csordas maintains that the subject/object distinction is not tenable when prioritizing perceptions and practices. The indeterminacy and flux inherent in cultural participation means it is not possible to delineate or isolate cultural objects or selves in the absence of social context, as they are constituted through experience.

The self has been repeatedly shown by anthropologists to be culturally constituted and qualitatively variable in place and time, as well as from culture to culture. Rather than being individual, it is sometimes *dividual* (divisible), as in the case of the Cuna Indians of Panama, who "say they have eight selves, each associated with a different part of the body" (Scheper-Hughes and Lock 1987:15). Western studies of human experience and behavior reflect a continual struggle with the inherent dualisms of Western forms of awareness, reflection, analysis, and discourse, which inevitably inform, often unconsciously and generally quite subtly, the perceptual and analytical efforts of anthropologists, sociologists, psychologists, neuroscientists, and other scholars concerned with human behavior. To live in the world means to repeatedly encounter ourselves and many others, people and places, the meanings of words, the flow of time, as well as powers of spirits, slogans, and popular ideologies. An infant's growth into a social person happens through gradual experience, by taking in the tastes, touching the textures, inhaling the smells, viewing the sights, and walking the walks of the world in which we are born, as well as those worlds that we encounter in our travels and relocations, be they willing or unwilling. Most of the time we take our perceptions and our classificatory schemes much for granted, as external, objective events and categories of perception that exist somehow beyond the ephemeral moment. A mind–body dualism has pervaded clinical sciences since before Hippocrates, while Descartes's larger than life intellectual inheritance has hegemonically defined the body's cognitive and sensory condition, being embedded in the modern biological art of seeing at the most physical level; in this linear light our bodies may be described as a kind of casing, a receiver or interface with the abundant natural/cultural world we inhabit, the mind hovering somewhere inside or beyond its edgy impermeable contours, waiting for messages to come through the brain.

In anthropology and the medical professions, scholars and clinicians have been struggling to adopt a more integrated perspective of health, illness, and suffering, but it is difficult to overcome the legacy and biases of dualistic, materialistic, and individualistic thinking, which are at the core of Western epistemologies and enmeshed with capitalist modes of production (Scheper-Hughes and Lock 1987:10, 22). Michel Foucault (1994 [1973]) has established the centrality of the body as an object of domination and a key site for the dialectic of power and knowledge, speaking of the descriptive act of medical science as "a seizure of being," an active way of shaping perception and creating new forms of knowledge and subjectivity. Social scientists, natural scientists, philosophers, and clinicians are finding that profoundly biased assumptions about the nature of people and the workings of bodies underlie authoritative writings and practices that are represented as fact or evidence-based in biomedical sciences and psychology: the assumption that individuation is a universal and necessary feature of human development, when in fact it is a recent development in Western societies, traceable to the late seventeenth century (not yet ingrained in Japan, where family and group loyalties supersede the individual as fundamental social units); the notion that personality dissociation and the experience of multiple selves is inherently pathological (not so in communities that practice shamanism or spirit possession); the concern with alienation in the arena of mental health, reflecting a predominantly Western social experience, tied to industrialization.

Embracing "the mindful body" proposed by Lock and Scheper-Hughes (1987) means recognizing the multifaceted non-dualism of embodied experience and allowing bodies a distinctly honored status and leading role in mapping of reality and the performance of healing: the mindful body is the existential and phenomenological basis of (a fullness of) self and social personhood, essential locus for sensation, participation, emotion, identity, and transformative experiences. I would add that the soulful body and the sensuous body deserve equally attentive, nuanced anthropological attention, beyond the well-established role of bodies as perceptual and cognitive agents, social symbols, or political instruments, which are inscribed, disciplined, segmented, or legislated in the field of power relations. As Renato Rosaldo (1989:39) observed: "If ideology often makes cultural facts appear natural, social analysis attempts to reverse the process." There is a taken-for-grantedness about the risks and options that we encounter, to use Emily Martin's (1994) words, a familiarity that people in developed societies learn through enculturation, education, media exposure, and many everyday experiences, a comfort that quickly vanishes when one stops to question and map routinized categories of understanding. In her provocative work *Flexible Bodies,* Emily Martin teases out the implications of the recent love affair with flexibility in American culture and how its language and imagery might have come to pervade "immunophilosophy" and the immunological descriptions of the body, late twentieth-century economic narratives on flexible specialization, production, and response to markets, human resources, organizations, or advertising. Like immunity, business success has become contingent on flexibility, not loyalty (Martin 1994:145).

Vision has long dominated the other senses in Western cultures. While most humans perceive more than a million colors, a few rare genetic variants supply an extra color-detecting cone in the retina, allowing the bearer to see 100 million colors, endowing those individuals with the perceptual abilities rivaling those of birds and reptiles (Roth 2006). But it is primarily our cultural experiences and interactions that influence what we recognize, what we remember, and what we are willing or able to describe in words or images. Biocultural understanding of vision and color has been most recently enhanced by brain imaging technologies (fMRI) and a surge in neuroscientific and psychological research on synesthesia: a "crosswiring" of sense perceptions, like the ability to associate colors with letters or with numbers, or see numbers as shapes or odors, which occurs in less than 5 percent of people. This sensory phenomenon appears to enhance memory and to be more prevalent in artists and highly creative people, such as physicist Richard Feynman. While there is a genetic basis, it is possible that everyone is born synesthetic to some degree, but brain connections undergo pruning as children mature and as environmental and cultural influences channel our perceptual abilities (Spector and Maurer 2009).

Western senses have been morphed and muffled through hundreds (or thousands) of years, from Plato to Descartes and Spinoza, through the disciplinary practices of empires and colonial regimes, the injunctions of manifold moralities (Catholic, Victorian, Protestant), the popular trends and social institutions that promoted particular regimes of perception and aesthetics (such as the Puritan view of bright colored clothing or the elitist view of folk painting as primitive and animalistic) all the way through the capitalist culture of consumption, which is enmeshed with the culture of "unorthodox medicine" and globalization. The sensescapes, desires, values, and practices of contemporary life are increasingly determined and informed by the ubiquity of the visual media. With the new hegemony of texting among the younger generations, we can add to this socio-sensory specialization the rise of communications that exclude most other sensory capacities from involvement to privilege just one or two of our sensory abilities. As we try to "capture a picture" of other cultures, with the recognition that it cannot be still and unchanging (like the putatively objective descriptions of early anthropologists), but a contingent, personal, and moving picture, we must remember how much of "the lived and the living" dimensions of human experience written words and captured images must inevitably omit, as it is all too easy to mistake our text and picture for reality itself.

Thus rises the call for an anthropology of embodiment, sensuous scholarship, and an anthropology of the senses involving fuller sensory participation, awareness, and presentation of ethnographic encounters, striving to give voice to native experiences rather than translating them in abstractions, to fully capture and flesh out the sensory experiences and embodied understandings of the people anthropologists aim to know. Whether awakening to the crowing of a flesh-and-bones rooster or the recorded "nature sounds" of a digital alarm clock, surrounded by the ripe, almost palpable pungency and thickness of farm odors, or the "fresh" synthetic and sanitized aromas of an urban condo, everyday sensory interaction and participation are the living ground where formative experiences of self emerge: the earliest preferences and tastes, social affinities, group identities, embodied and often unconscious orientations to the values of material, ideological, and cultural worlds that humans inhabit. Marcel Mauss (1990 [1950, 1925]) referred to the body as "the first and most natural tool of man." Mary Douglas (1970) explored centrality of the body among natural symbols. English language idioms of power relationships such as "saving face," "putting one's foot in one's mouth," being "the right arm" or "the right hand" of a powerful person, or "head-hunting" in the corporate world capture the primary role of embodied experiences for self and social interaction, bodies serving as maps in negotiating who we are and how we relate with others. Rituals such as communion through bread-as-body-of-Christ similarly evoke how the body serves to enmesh us socially and spiritually into particular traditions.

The Anthropology of Sensations and the Multidimensionality of Healing Work

A clear distinction between cognitive, emotional, and physical experiences or sensations is not made similarly in all cultures, although it is a common fact of communication in Western settings and particularly relevant for health care. When working among the Anlo people of Ghana, anthropologist Kathryn Linn Geurts (2002) found that her model of the five senses could not be neatly matched with local categories of perception and awareness. The local term *seselelame* "straddles that supposed divide" between cognitive perception and physical sensation, being at various time used to mean hearing, tasting, smelling, understanding, obeying, sexual arousal, heartache, passion, the inspiration to dance or speak, or a tingling of the skin that may indicate impending illness (Geurts 2002:41). Geurts has suggested that *seselelame* is a kind of synesthetic "metasense" that provides a basis for organizing embodied experience and comprehending the world in Anlo culture, which is fundamentally different from the organ-based model of five senses used in Western cultures. Furthermore, she argues that, while it appears to be an objective scientific reality, verified by medicine and psychology, the five-sense model is a "folk ideology": recent scientific research with animals, humans, and robots indicates that there are more senses than just five (Geurts 2002:228–30). The Anlo-Ewe language and culture provide terms for fifty "kinesthetic styles" of walking, which reflect the person's moral character.

The definitions and research agenda pertaining to a new "anthropology of sensations" have been rigorously laid out as a field of study in a recent seminal article by Devon Hinton, David Howes, and Laurence Kirmayer, who note that "the processes of selective filtering and the organization of sensations into meaningful perceptions are of particular relevance to the anthropology of medicine and a number of authors have stressed the importance of attending to sensations in studying the illness experience" (2008:143). Following a recent trend of merging neurophysiology with anthropology, phenomenology, and psychology, the authors define "sensations" as faculties of physical perception, noting that they were once called "wits," and that the five senses may actually be anywhere from four to eight, but that "any division of the nervous system that provides information about the state of the body or the surrounding environment to the brain, which reaches some level of consciousness, is a 'sense'" (Hinton et al. 2008:143).

Hinton, Howes, and Kirmayer (2008:144) offer a provisional list of eleven sense types that includes visual (sight), auditory (hearing), olfactory (smell), gustatory (taste), proprioceptive-kinesthetic (limb and muscle position), vestibular (head movement) muscle and tendon tension, gastrointestinal distention, temperature, skin pressure, oxygen, and carbon dioxide level (which may cause shortness of breath). Sensations arise from the senses and may also "arise from sensorial blends" of multiple senses; thus one may categorize them further as monomodal and polymodal. Highly relevant in health care are polymodal sensations such as dizziness, nausea, pain, heart motions, and shortness of breath, which can originate in one or a variety of combinations of the sense types.

Of anthropological interest and relevance are the diverse ways in which sensations are experienced and labeled cross-culturally. Six tastes are recognized in India, rather than four, for example. Cultures recognize different qualities and abilities as significant, providing terminology, guidance, and reinforcement for discriminating those features that are deemed important. The authors note that each culture, person, or time in history may have specific "forms of sensation experience" as complex loops connect cultural categories and modes of perception with physiology, attention, and imagination; among the ways and "mechanisms for generating and amplifying sensations" they describe:

- attention: focusing on particular sensation in a particular area of the body
- anxiety and depression: causing increased brain reactivity to stimuli and changes in the autonomic nervous system, with experiences such as cold extremities
- cultural syndromes: culturally specific patterns of distress that include ideas about causation, symptoms, or remedies; that is, *susto* (or fright sickness) in South America
- ethnophysiology: local concepts and concerns about organs and body processes, such as concern with the abdomen in Japan or the heart in the United States (Lock 1980)
- external stimuli: such as sensitivity to particular sensory inputs based on the meaning attributed to the stimulus and its relation to the state of the person
- imagination: including attention, anxiety, and percept flashbacks (revisiting)
- metaphor: inducing sensations by metaphorical means, often polymodal
- self-image: sensations feeding into particular self-images (i.e., flexible, burdened)
- sensation kindling: repeated experiencing can create an easily activated neural circuit that increases the susceptibility to the sensation from other causes
- traumatic memory: evoking specific memories that cause sensations, such as "somatic flashbacks" (Hinton et al. 2008:147–52)

Hinton, Howes, and Kirmayer (2008:153) say that sensations can trigger or anchor particular scripts, but sensory experience is also malleable, allowing new meanings and associations to be created. This the authors recognize as the basis for the transformations of experience that healing practices can bring about. If one of my happiest memories is swinging in a large wooden swing at my grandmother's house, swinging in such a swing will reactivate that sense of joy; at the same time, I can replay that memory in my head at times when I need comfort, strength, or reassurance. Healing can entail sensations (as well as images and stories), note the authors, "that invoke a script that increases a sense of efficacy and promotes positive engagement in the life process." For transformative change to occur, there must be shifts in "embodied metaphor, memory and self-image": sensations are *key sites* for these processes, as bodily sensations contribute vivid imagery to communication (such as calling someone "a pain in the neck"), play an instrumental role in memory making (we tend to remember being slapped or caressed or the sweetness of watermelons), and a major contributor to our sense of who we are (such as "I am run down and getting old, because my joints hurt"); these elements are particularly influential in relation to traumatic experiences. Scripting and rescripting can be therapeutic.

Excellent examples of this come from birthing: women's cultural ideas of birth greatly influence their perception and interpretation of pain in childbirth. Cecilia Van Hollen (2003) explored South Indian women's acceptance of oxytocin-induced birthing and resistance to anesthesia, noting both their distinctive embodiment and interpretation of pain and modern technologies of reproduction and how these were elaborately interwoven with issues of power, gender, and postcolonial development. Anne Fadiman's account of Hmong birthing notes that women would traditionally give birth alone, without a sound, and that their stoic demeanor did not endear them to the hospital staff in California, as they would often arrive there in very late stages of labor; thus they dubbed wheelchairs "Hmong birthing chairs" because sometimes they did not make it all the way to the delivery room. Additionally, Hmong have a deep antipathy toward the practices of blood drawing (as it is believed to be limited) and anesthesia (as it separates the soul from the body), and are resistant to a number of common biomedical interventions. In her detailed account of the home birthing movement, Klassen describes the ways in which American women of diverse faiths (Jewish, Christian, Muslim, etc.) empower themselves through home birthing experiences, embracing pain, as they negotiate their feminine and spiritual aspirations. The home birth movement and the resurgence of midwifery in the United States is a phenomenon that has been gaining momentum since the 1960s and that has been much aided by the influential work and activism of anthropologists, particularly Brigitte Jordan and Robbie Davis-Floyd, who helped to fissure the technocratic model of hospital birth, in which women's knowledge and intuition were systematically denied and silenced. Jordan (1992) described the honored role of Maya midwives, the tradition of regular home visits, examination, and massage given by the midwife to the pregnant woman, and the ability of midwives to turn breech babies, a procedure that many modern ob/gyn doctors do not have experience performing.

Smell and Taste

The body knows the world through odors, flavors, sounds, colors, touch, pain, and the rhythms of cultural routines and revelries, but it is the sense of smell that provides a most direct link to the brain, through the olfactory nerve. Studies have shown that a newborn infant clearly recognizes a breast-pad impregnated with her mother's breastmilk among those impregnated with the milk of other mothers, pointing to the powerful survival and evolutionary meaning of smell. Constance Classen (1992:133) rightly noted that people tend be accustomed to their own odors, but notice the odors of others. The Dassantech people of Ethiopia provide a striking illustration of what Classen calls "olfactory class divisions," as they are divided into pastoralists and fishermen, the former being regarded as superior, and they identify themselves by the odor of their environment. Everything associated with cattle is considered good and good-smelling, while the odor of fish and fishermen is considered by the pastoralists to be foul. Strict social barriers are upheld by the herders, who interact only minimally with the "other" group. Classen suggests that the repugnance felt by the pastoralists is a reaction to the social threat of disorder and symbolically grounded in the notion of fish as anomalous with regards to the cycles of nature: their reproduction seems acyclical and their smell is said to persist indefinitely.

The smell of women is commonly classified as foul in societies where the status of women is low, with different responses toward different aspects and categories of femininity. Whereas the smell of young and fertile women is often described as pleasant, menstruation is perceived as smelly and polluting in many cultures, including premodern Europe, where it could spoil fertility, and the Pacific Islands, where it could impair men's hunting abilities. Not coincidentally, Classen (1992:142) observes that the smell of prostitutes and morally loose women is considered distasteful, illustrated by the Spanish term *puta*, which originates in the Latin word for putrid. Moreover, in the Western popular imagination, witches and enchantresses are associated with sweet, evil scents, as echoed by fragrance names such as "Black Magic" and "Poison" (Classen 1992:144). As mentioned earlier, the witch represents a social threat as a marginal person who undermines the social order and the power of men.

The amount of body odor also varies according to the number of sweat glands one possesses, with some racial/ethnic groups sweating a lot more than others and varying degrees of tolerance and appreciation for natural bodily smells. More than any other culture, however, Western cultures attempt to remove and cover up bodily and environmental odors. Foreign-born people living in the United States are often perceived as alien-smelling, either wearing too much cologne or not wearing enough deodorizers, depending on their culture of origin. Like other animals, humans secrete pheromones to attract the opposite sex. During ovulation, hormonal changes also produce changes in body odor among most mammal species, including humans. It is ironic that smells such as musk, which originates in a gland of the musk deer, is diluted for use in perfumery, even though it is repulsive at full strength. While signifying the wilderness, power, and "otherness" of nature, it is also a means to symbolically appropriate those powers (Classen 1992:46).

Likewise, the pungency of plants, herbs, and spices used for cooking and healing, while unpleasant to some, at least initially, serve to create familiarity and reinforce cultural identities. The comforting smell of cinnamon during winter holidays or chicken soup on a cold winter night refract much deeper cultural schemas and scripts of relationship and community. Ethnic groups have very strong attraction and revulsion to the smells of traditional foods and spices. Our senses inform us of threats and boundaries and smells are among the most powerful triggers of emotion, desire, and repulsion; thus the metaphoric expressions of "smelling a fear," or the phrase "smelling a rat" for sensing betrayal or deceit. In contrast to the upsetting and immoral connotations of decay, the bodies of saints and the divine are associated with the emanations of beautiful odors. The use of smells for celebration, relaxation, and healing has been documented cross-culturally and is further explored in this chapter in the discussion of aromatherapy.

In his work on taste, Bourdieu (1984) focused on the "sense of taste" as a key organizing principle of experience, aesthetics, and social life, showing how the human ability to discriminate flavors and express preferences is embedded and enmeshed in the social fabric, linked with issues of identity and social class. We depend on our senses to guide and nourish our imaginations as we struggle to apprehend the beauty, value, and meaning of things around us. We reach toward the ripe apple, feel its slight globular body, and then grab the fruit's eerily smooth, firm skin with our fingertips, work in a slight sniff, and then pull away ever so briefly to examine its color and skin with small brown freckles before sinking all our teeth into it, letting that juicy sweetness dribble down the chin. The role of taste in human history and power relations cannot be understated: from ambrosia and nectar to beer and wine, to the spices of the East, salt, coffee, sugar, cocoa, and most recently corn syrup, the myriad flavors of the earth have conquered and transformed the world of humans just as much as humans have transformed theirs (Mintz 1985; Pollan 2006).

Taste, like smell, provides a powerful metaphor for experience—bitter cold, sour face, sweet revenge, taste of success, taste of blood, or getting a taste of your own medicine—such idioms are reminders of the intimacy of taste, which is the only one of the five "official" senses that entails bringing the object inside the body, or more accurately, inside the head. The sense of taste has been historically considered one of the "lower" senses and gluttony has been associated with animality, which in turn has been contrasted with the higher faculties and senses, concerned with philosophy and art. It is true, however, that the sense of taste used to be more likely to be involved in excessive consumption. Urinotherapy (the practice of drinking one's own urine) is supposed to have the most profound healing effects imaginable, as it symbolically represents a self-sufficiency and self-renewal, having had deep roots in the Indian subcontinent as well as advocates on every continent, including North America. Tasting and eating the self is in fact the polar opposite of cannibalism, which is known to have been practiced to ceremonially honor or incorporate the power and identity of the "other." At the same time, taste is the most honored sense because it partakes of Holy Communion; the supreme and sublime Christian act of sacramental worship is symbolic transgression, since it represents eating and drinking the body and the blood of the divine being.

It is very telling of human nature that taste is said to "be acquired" (preferences are learned) and that it is used as a marker for aesthetic sophistication, as people judge one another and cultural products as to whether they are in "good taste" or "bad taste." When we are born, we quickly acquire a preference for sweetness, like the mother's milk, and it is not long before babies begin to spit out foods that are unfamiliar. Some even refuse solid food, developing an aversion to it, if not introduced around six or eight months of age. Trying to feed a baby for the first time or offering a new food is inevitably both frustrating and comical, especially witnessing a sudden but unmistakable expression of disgust triggered by a new food. If we accidentally put something in the mouth and do not recognize the taste, or find something odd about the texture of the food, there is an instant compulsion to spit it out.

Plato identified the four principal tastes as bitter, sour (acid), sweet, and salty, adding also harsh, astringent, and pungent, and Aristotle attempted to connect them to the seven basic colors (Korsmeyer 2002:14). The ability to discriminate taste is an important adaptation, since plants in their race for survival tend to signal their poisonous (often medicinal) properties through bitter tasting chemicals, which would discourage predatory action. It is also adaptive for toddlers to go through a "picky phase," since in a hunter and gatherer environment, it was essential for survival for the child to avoid untested foods and eat preferentially what the mother was eating, to avoid sickness, nausea, or poisoning. Whereas it seems fairly common to classify taste in terms of limited cultural categories, it is important to keep in mind that people also respond quite discriminately to texture, which can be argued to be yet another mouth sense. The term "mouth feel" is an important notion in product-testing and marketing of food and wine. Interestingly, the ability to discriminate among numerous wines and beers suggests that the possibilities of taste may be much misrepresented linguistically. A national and global trend toward high-carbohydrate, high-salt foods compels us to eat more and more, with minimal nutrient content and less variety. Overconsumption of sweets is well documented to have increased drastically in this century, with dire health effects.

Taste also plays an important role in learning and memory. In Marcel Proust's remarkable work *The Remembrance of Things Past*, the journey back in time is triggered by the taste of a Petite Madeleine, a small cake that is served with coffee. Saying that something left a bad taste in one's mouth describes the difficulty of forgetting a bad experience. More so than every other sensory capability, taste signifies an experience of deep intimacy, of internalizing or being a part of something or becoming part of a community. Eating and drinking together is one of the most fundamental acts of sociality and connection, just like the refusal of food when it is being offered is cross-culturally considered to be disrespectful, if not offensive. At the same time, eating is governed at least in part by taboos and rituals that seek to restrain the senses either permanently or periodically, such as the refusal to eat meat exemplified by members of the Brahmin (priestly) caste in India or by Catholic Christians during Lent. In recent decades, there has been a growing awareness of the ways in which capitalist environments overstimulate the senses in the interests of marketing and consumer satisfaction and local movements have emerged to challenge the *fast-foodisme* of mass consumption (Howes 2005:297). Eating is a dynamic expression of identity politics.

According to Paul Stoller (1997:47), in Mali and Niger, "Songhay sorcerers eat power," an act that can both empower and overpower their bodies; they also "eat history," thus becoming "owned" by the "old words" they have ingested. Adeline Masquelier (2001) has woven a vibrant and complex account of Mawri women's experiences: their ritual relationships to the spirit world, their daily struggles with health, money, and relationships, and the intimate and pervasive impact of consumer culture. Notably, for these enterprising Mawri women of Niger, the metaphor of sweetness ably connects the domains of prostitution, childbirth, and the dangers of excessive consumption.

Tactile Experiences

The beneficial effects of touch and massage have been amply documented since antiquity. The benefits of skin-to-skin contact extend from the prolonged and intimate bonding of infants with their caregivers and pregnancy massage to "bonesetting" and other kinds of body work practiced in societies worldwide. Over the past thirty years, numerous scientific studies with premature infants and full-term infants and toddlers have demonstrated that infants who received massage and skin-to-skin contact left the neonatal ICU sooner, gained more weight (as much as 20 percent more per day), slept better, and had better neurological development. One of the measures used to determine decrease in stress levels is the level of the adrenal hormone *cortisol*, which reliably decreases as a result of touch-based thereapies. Touch Research Institute (TRI) at the University of Miami School of Medicine studies show similar benefits in cocaine-exposed preterm babies, as well as stressed babies; fathers who massaged their babies for fifteen minutes daily for a month were more expressive and showed more warmth during play; massage with oil had a more pronounced calming effect than massage without oil (TRI 2011).

Two healing traditions that can be considered success stories in the arena of "manual medicine" are osteopathy and chiropractic medicine, which have been able to establish themselves solidly as professionalized medical systems, reimbursed by insurance companies in the United States and elsewhere. Since its beginnings in the late nineteenth century, when its founder called himself a "bonesetter" and believed that the manipulation of bones could correct imbalances and blockages in one's vital fluid, osteopathy has departed most notably from its beginnings: its primary reliance on physical manipulation and realignment taking a back seat to mainstream methods of care (Gevitz 1988). Osteopathy has nearly merged with biomedical practice in the United States, adopting fairly standard biomedical criteria of legitimization, equivalent programs of study, and nearly identical methods. Thus, it cannot be considered as a genuine "alternative" practice anymore. Chiropractic has also become integrated in Western health care systems, although maintaining secondary status as a "heterodox" approach; the premises, the safety, and the effectiveness of chiropractic continue to be questioned and challenged by medical doctors and physical therapists, despite its popularity. Because of the current congruence of osteopathy and chiropractic with the predominantly mechanistic style of mainstream medicine, and because their histories and practices have become widely known and documented as they have resurged in popularity, I will not explore them further here.

Detailed accounts of both professions are included in numerous recent books on leading forms of CAM and integrative medicine by historians, sociologists, and anthropologists, including in the works of Hans Baer, Waltraud Ernst, James Whorton, and Norman Gevitz.

Dorothea Hover-Kramer is a holistic nurse and educator who played an instrumental role in the development of the healing touch (HT) method of channeling energy healing through the hands, together with Janet Mentgen and Susan Morales, creating a specific curriculum and program that supports learners in a long-term way. They point to a long history of energy use in medicine (x-rays, magnets, and more recently, electricity-based pain relief), the body being an energy system. Hover-Kramer (2002:16) contends that brain waves of healers in the healing act are all around 8 hertz, resonating the earth's electromagnetic field. Healing touch practitioners use the seven chakras, energy vortices along the spine, each governing particular physical, emotional, mental, and spiritual functions, and each being associated with a particular color, together with a four-layer model of the body's energy field: (1) vital layer or etheric field, (2) emotional layer or aura, (3) mental or causal layer, and (4) intuitive or astral field (Hover-Kramer 2002:69). This model was also the basis for another influential healing system, therapeutic touch (TT), developed a few years earlier by Dora Kunz and Dr. Dolores Krieger (1979) at New York University. Healing touch practice benefits a wide array of conditions, including stress and cardiovascular problems, back problems, arthritis, depression, abuse, and autoimmune dysfunctions. Both Hover-Kramer and Krieger have written about altered states of consciousness and transformations experienced by healers who become empowered and sensitized to their bodily perceptions through practices of "centering" and energy manipulation, such as smoothing and ruffling the fields. There are visible signs of the relaxation response in the person receiving healing.

Glyn Adams (2002) described his experience as a student and practitioner of shiatsu in Britain, comparing it to the way shiatsu has been practiced in Japan, its country of origin. Reflecting on how lung function was presented at a weekend seminar at the British School of Shiatsu-Do, Adams noted that the presentation reflected a Traditional Chinese Medicine perspective. Governed by the metal element, lungs control *ki* energy and respiration, channels and blood vessels, water passages, hair and skin, as well as representing "a physical border between a person's self and the world beyond" (Adams 2002:252). The role of the lungs was consistent with earlier anthropological work on China, but the psychological interpretations offered by the students in Britain reflected New Age notions of the autonomous person. Less than two hundred years old, Western individualism is the ground for an autonomous search for self-realization, including reflexive ways of living that replace external moral guidelines with self-reflection and integration of various aspects of the self (mind, body, spirit) aimed at achieving a more genuine and meaningful life. This is a modern quest and a key aspect of the New Age movement, quite distinct from the traditional Japanese notion of personhood, which is socio-centric. Based on earlier

work in Japan, such as Lock's (1980), Adams suggests that relief from illness en-
compasses both a resolution of social disharmony and "bodily holism," which entails
attention to diet and well-being without necessarily engaging with patients' personal
circumstances directly. Participation into a client's project of self-care as a project of
spiritual and moral growth is a distinctive feature of New Age healing.

Adams notes that tactile experience involves "a system of differentiated therapeutic touch" in response to the clients' particular needs and concerns, as they are
sensed and interpreted by the practitioner, creating "an opportunity for reflexive
self-engagement that constitutes 'healing,'" and that "touch has distinct metaphorical potential" (2002:261). Adopting a phenomenological approach, which seeks to
capture the immediacy of embodied knowledge that precedes academic schemes and
interpretations, Adams provides a nuanced and illuminating description of a particular therapeutic episode to show how "differing holisms animate the worlds of a
practitioner and client" (2002:255). In tending to Jane, a married woman in her 60s
with neck and shoulder discomfort and anxiety (a common profile for seekers of
body-work therapies) Adams describes "feeling" Jane's neck as tense and her chest
as weak, along with a disturbance of boundary permeability that he recognized as a
metal imbalance—so he decided to use a "metal touch" to work on Jane's "embodied
boundaries." The account goes back and forth between the practitioner's own sensory engagement in the experience of providing treatment and Jane's response to the
treatment, including his own relaxation and a sense of emptiness, the awareness of
resistance to certain attempted motions of shoulder rotation, to which he responds by
giving up expectations, remembering "that metal touch meant working with boundaries sensitively" (Adams 2002:258). The practitioner adapted the movements ac-
cordingly, using palpable descriptions such as "I listened with my hands into Jane's
shoulder," to discover that Jane is becoming deeply relaxed. Adams writes:

> Moving along the base of the neck with my thumb and focusing into my belly, I imagined
> I was sitting supported by a large balloon. My thumb sank deeply into the acupuncture
> point Gall Bladder 12, slowly sinking through layers of skin, fascia, muscle, to reach
> bone at the point's base. I made small, slow circles with my thumb and the supporting
> hand, tracing a figure eight for a minute or two. Moving on to the next point, I experi-
> enced the same sense of emptiness; these points were *kyo,* I reflected. (2002: 258)

He was surprised to feel a profound sense of calm, warmth, and buoyancy, along
with a feeling of buzzing in his thumb, while at the same time noticing a change
in the air of the room, which gained "a strange, sticky, glutinous quality" (Adams
2002:259). As he worked on Jane's neck, the therapist describes that the boundaries
between his hands and her neck became fluid, and he felt the need to do less and
less, not knowing who was directing the movements, unexpectedly losing "a normal
sense of separateness," and then noticing that "the area around Jane's neck seemed
light and alive" (Adams 2002:259).

Later, Jane shared her experience as having sensed two comforting spirits in the room, including a "Chinaman," sitting in the corner as her guide, drawing upon her acquaintance with spiritualist teachings that identified the neck area as an entry point for healing energies (Adams 2002:260). It is significant that while the therapist interpreted his experience of "embodied confluence" as stemming from the state of points, forces, and meridians in Jane's shoulders derived from the ethnophysiology of TCM, the client sharing the powerful therapeutic experience interpreted it in her own spiritualist framework. The author notes that since returning from an extended visit to Japan, "feelings of deep stillness" occur to him often and do not seem unusual anymore. Drawing on a model of personhood, bodily function, etiology, and therapeutic action that blended elements of TCM, shiatsu, and New Age, Adams suggests that the physical and emotional boundaries associated with the metal element were manifested in the full stretch of the arm as an embodied boundary. Using various learned techniques of touch on her neck, Adams expresses his "embodied intention to suggest an embodied permeability to Jane," which may further work on a client's psychological boundaries within minutes, hours, or days of treatments, conjuring the possibility that:

> the suggestion of an embodied permeability might also potentially lead to changes in a client's pre-reflexive embodied sense of self, namely the aspect of the self engaged with the world in ways that are distinct from rational, interpretive modes of reflection. (2002:261)

Adams's vivid description of the therapeutic encounter in the context of a British shiatsu therapeutic modality ties into the manifold mechanisms of amplifying sensation described by Hinton, Howes, and Kirmayer, most notably directing *attention* to sensations, aptly evoked in his account; *imagination*, as expressed in the therapist's image of sitting on a large balloon, the increased viscosity of the air, or the client's visualization of healing spirits; *ethnophysiology,* represented by the energy points and forces perceived by the healer; the use of metaphors to direct awareness such as "metal touch"; and the experience of *sensation kindling*, documented by Adams's comment that the deep stillness experience, surprising at first, became common through continued practice and journeying to Japan.

Rhythm, Movement, and Music as Life

It takes about forty weeks of prenatal development before an infant can smell, taste, touch, or see the outside world firsthand. But quite some time before birth, fetuses become able to feel the rocking motion of the mother's walking and the constant, muffled sound of her heartbeat through the watery, pear-shaped cocoon. Because human babies are born more helpless than other mammals, it takes nine more months, after the nine months inside the womb, for a baby and mother to begin to comfortably separate for brief periods, as long as they are in a secure environment. In most traditional cultures, like the !Kung or the Gusii, babies are held most of the time by a kin-person. In many places they are swaddled and tied to the mother in a sling as she works the land, a practice that has reemerged and been dubbed "kangaroo care," and which has been proven to give beneficial stimulation and comfort to babies, providing notable benefit to premature and colicky infants. Most babies like to be rocked or vibrated gently, undoubtedly a reminder of life in the womb, experiencing a soothing, pleasurable stimulation to the inner ear.

Scientific studies have confirmed that even before they are born, babies recognize their mother's voice and respond to music. The early attunement to (and recognition of) the distinctive sounds of the native language has also been demonstrated, with young infants sucking more actively on a pacifier when hearing familiar sounds. That sounds and music are so appealing to infants explains the universal existence of lullabies, some with fairly bizarre lyrics, which probably expressed the parent's sleepless frustration at 4:00 A.M. In capitalist consumer society, the cohabiting grandmother has been supplanted with an array of vibrating rockers and musical toys. As a result of studies that suggested a beneficial effect of music on the development of intelligence, known as "the Mozart effect," the market has been inundated with recordings especially for babies, some even for babies to listen to in the womb, with headphones pressed against the mother's belly. The consensus is, however, that the effect is not limited to Mozart or classical music but that many other types of melodious music can be beneficial as well: the experience of clearly patterned musical sounds and early exposure to music seems to be connected with superior performance on other right-brain tasks, such as mathematics. In most people the right brain is the site for emotions, dreams, visual-spatial skills, body image, and awareness (Joseph 1988). However, more recent studies using technologies such as fMRI paint a more complex picture of music in the human brain, showing that while listening mostly resides in the right hemisphere, the activities of musicians make significant use of their left hemisphere. The brain has a property called plasticity: the ability to change and adapt organization, depending on experience.

A recent neuroscience article by Salimpoor et al. (2011) documents the existence of "anatomically distinct dopamine release during anticipation and experience of peak emotion in music," intense pleasure being mediated by the mesolimbic system, which is involved in motivation and reinforcement. The authors note tongue-in-cheek that food, psychoactive drugs, and money are also stimuli that generate such pleasure. It seems puzzling for scientists that this same pathway is involved for less tangible things like music and art (seemingly not considered essential to survival in an immediate way), especially since both cultural and individual preferences play a significant role in the response to these abstract stimuli. It is interesting to note here how all this comes full circle: leading anthropologists of shamanism have been tapping into recent neuroscience insights to argue for the evolutionary and social value of ASCs and group rituals on the basis that they promote brain integration and activate the limbic system while regulating the autonomic nervous systems and healing many states of stress or distress. Traditional rituals are always associated with repetitive sounds (made by clapping, shaking a rattle, or rhythmic drumming) and very often involve rhythmic movement or dance. The synergy of these experiences makes rituals a powerful emotional experience and brings about an emotional release, traditionally referred to as *catharsis*. It is no coincidence that the Hindu word *raga* means both music and mood, designating a dazzling spectrum of traditional musical forms, capturing highly specific moods and emotions through structured improvisation. *Ragas* are sometimes used as homeopathic remedies.

Psychotherapists have had success in treating diverse mental and emotional problems with voice therapy and mindfulness exercises, which can induce a deep state of relaxation and integration even without movement. The Sanskrit syllable *om* is considered a representation of the divine and a means of union with the divine. When uttered as a group, for example, in a yoga class, it resonates throughout the group creating a most extraordinary sense of peaceful communion. A comparable practice is used in the Orthodox Christian tradition of monasticism: the rhythmic repetition of the Prayer of the Heart or the utterance of the Lord's Prayer in conjunction with focused breathing and proper posture are known to facilitate gnostic experiences, visions of the uncreated light of the beginning, and ultimately *theosis*—personal communion with the Divinity. Dance therapy, along with a variety of movement-based therapies like Alexander Technique and Contact Improv, has been successfully used in Western societies for decades, sometimes in conjunction with other forms of therapy, including music, guided imagery, and creative visualization. Whether moving alone, in step, or entwined together with someone in a tango embrace, the experience of dance is powerfully emotional and communal.

More than any one element taken in isolation, the synesthetic combination of breath, sound, and movement is extremely powerful, its central role in traditional healing practices worldwide representing its evolutionary significance for integrating human consciousness, synchronizing mental processes, and promoting psychosocial well-being. The understanding and acceptance of synesthetic healing is expanding in biomedical circles as neuroscience is able to validate the benefits of these practices and experiences by making them visible and thus more "real" by Western standards. Recent studies published in the *New England Journal of Medicine* suggest possible beneficial effects of tai chi for fibromyalgia. Others document benefits for heart disease, arthritis, fall prevention, and cancer survivors (Brown 2010). The medicinal benefits of mindful movement are advocated by Peter Wayne, PhD, founder and director of the Tree of Life Tai Chi Center in Boston, assistant professor of medicine at Harvard Medical School, and director of the Tai Chi/Mind-Body Research Program at Harvard Medical School's Osher Research Center. In the Osher Research Center lab, Wayne's colleague Catherine Kerr examines the effects of tai chi, qigong, mindfulness, and acupuncture on cortical dynamics and the sense of touch (Osher 2011).

Reflecting on a recent randomized controlled trial designed for the study of qigong, Kerr (2002) noted a discrepancy between the understandings and experiences of the researchers, who viewed it as a *non-specific* mind-body therapy for exercise and relaxation, and the qigong master's understanding of it as a *purposeful* "mind-in-body" therapy, in which certain movements and visualizations are used to focus attention on particular areas of the body. She pointed out that the qigong method is deeply embedded in Chinese notions of health and the body, and a culturally grounded interpretation of what bodily feelings mean (Kerr 2002:437). While the practitioner employs the "mind-in-the-belly" metaphor as a *real* experiential feeling, the researcher perceives it as being an expression of faith or a spiritual belief. Ultimately, the physiological and mental effects of such metaphors will vary greatly, depending on how the metaphors are embodied or "somatized" by participants. Since the way we inhabit our bodies is shaped by our cultures, our memories, and our emotions, not only our cognitive processes, mimicking the motions of qigong may not necessarily duplicate the experience. Distinct somatic modes of attention and different embodiments and feelings triggered by metaphors like "mind-in-the-belly" will produce different effects.

Dance and movement therapy have a long and diverse history worldwide, comprising professionalized, franchised, traditional, and indigenous forms and methodologies, from the most ancient to recent, hybrid, eclectic, trendy creations, such as Nia (nianow.com). Randall McClellan (1991) provided a detailed account of musical healing based on the Tantra Yoga chakra system, which links each one of the chakras (energy center situated along the spine) with a particular set of vowels, colors, and sound qualities that stimulate particular organs and endocrine glands. More recently, synesthetic connections between movement, music, and healing experiences have been explored in several important works, offering richly contextualized accounts of the therapeutic and transformative roles of music in non-Western societies, notably the influential work of Benjamin D. Koen (2009), Penelope Gouk (2000), and Marina Roseman (1993). The emergent field of medical ethnomusicology is distinguished by the recent publication of *The Oxford Handbook of Medical Ethnomusicology* (Koen et al. 2009).

Case Study: Becoming Radiant—Real Reiki in Postsocialist Romania

During my 1998 fieldwork in Romania I focused my attention on alternative healing movements, competing discourses on health, illness, and the body, and their relationship to social and historical circumstances of the Romanian "transition." I saw the powerful emergence of alternative medicines since the fall of the Ceauşescu dictatorship in 1989 as an effort to reconfigure the notions of the self, body, illness, and medical knowledge in a manner that opposed the biomedical model identified with the centralized state authority. I had envisioned the healing that people were seeking as a holistic effort to redefine the self and the body in the absence of communist authority and a centralized biomedical hierarchy. I had also hypothesized that the restoration of balance aimed at by alternative medical practices would be analogous to and symbolic of the repair which was hoped to take place in Romanian society.

The need for social healing in the aftermath of communism was illustrated in the words spoken in a February 26, 1998, interview on ProTV by Andrei Pleşu, a leading Romanian writer and scholar and Minister of External Affairs at the time of my fieldwork. Pleşu affirmed: "We are ill and we are legitimately ill. For decades there were all kinds of toxins injected upon us. Sometimes the recovery lasts longer than the illness. There are convalescences that leave you more run down than the illness itself." Economic and power inequities constituted an omnipresent and painful reality in postsocialist Romania, a state of disharmony within the social body.

During a conference I was introduced to Dora and Vlad, a two-person team of Radiant Technique instructors who had published several books on the subject. Radiant Technique is one of several distinct traditions of reiki practice, all of which trace their origins to Japan and to founder Dr. Mikao Usui through Dr. Barbara Rey. The basic level of this practice involves laying hands to allow vital energy to flow through the palms toward the desired site. The more advanced levels allow transmission of energy across time and space without physical contact. Once initiated in Radiant Technique (also called Real Reiki), one is referred to as a Radiant and becomes a "giver of light," the same energy form as love and prayer.

Dora and Vlad were people in their 40s, with scientific backgrounds. I attended their seminars, earning a first- and subsequently a second-degree diploma in Radiant Technique. The first session took place inside a tall apartment complex in one of Bucharest's newer, peripheral neighborhoods. There were fifteen other persons in the class, ranging in ages from 13 to over 60. Dora and Vlad described the ability of radiant touch as a natural ability of all living things and a quality that "belongs to the whole." Through a series of four secret "tunings" and by learning a sequence of powerful symbols, the trainee enters in resonance with the supreme principle of the universe. The instructors described the learning of and initiation into Radiant Technique as a process of awakening and conscientization. In their view, Radiant Technique is part of the "school of mysteries": based on the intuitive aspects of mind and on vibration, rather than information. They stressed that this approach is not a sect, religion, philosophical system, diagnosis method, massage technique, hypnosis, or self-hypnosis. Rather, it is a *science of universal energy*, with precise laws, established over time through experience. Dora spoke of approaching one's life as a work of art, embracing each person's uniqueness. In manifesting itself, the divinity was careful never to repeat itself. Underlying the diversity, there is a center, universal in character. Dora spoke melodiously: "God created life out of life, everything out of the divine being. God did not create anything that is dead." Seamlessly layering Orthodox Christianity with animistic beliefs, Dora asserted that stones also breathe, once in millennia. Minerals too are alive and connected to the Supreme Being.

Dora and Vlad drew a diagram of the energetic model of living things, human beings in particular: a series of seven concentric circles, numbered from 1, for the one
closest to the center, to 7, for the farthest and largest one. The first body is the physical body ("solid" or "matter"), a form of energy with low frequencies, of approximately 7Hz. This is the body on which the surgeon works, and it is the body to which
we tend to give the most attention. Yet it is only a part of our energetic structure,
according to the bioenergetic model of the body. Dora stressed that every level needs
nourishment and care (washing or purification or beautification), or it becomes like
the garden of a lazy gardener. The second body is the "emotional body," composed of
the sum of our sentiments and desires. It brightly colored, human-shaped, and con-
tinuously moving, like flames of a fire. The "mental body," our third layer, comprises
the multitude of one's thoughts: the rational mind. It is an instrumental level for work
"here on Earth." Dora affirmed that the thought always appears first, then the action
follows. She added: "In Genesis, the human being was created in the image of God.
Perfection is the purpose towards which we are headed. . . . Of all creatures on Earth,
only the human being was given the ability to co-create consciously with Divinity."

"What is our purpose or role here on Earth?" the instructors asked. People encounter many false ideas, illusions, and fantasies that can lead them down the wrong
path. An erroneous understanding of life or of the relationship with those around us
can create energetic stases and health problems as well, the teachers suggested. "The
body with higher vibration shapes the ones with lower vibrations. Thus, the majority
of illnesses and destinies are the result of the mental body." If one puts the acorn in
the ground and favorable conditions are given, an oak tree like the father oak will
grow, which can, in turn, pass on the same values. This is similar to the "seed of
light" placed by divinity in the human being, they said. Our virtues make this seed
develop. While there are other levels of the auras, these three levels—physical, emotional, and mental—are the most well-known ones. Medicine acts on all three, but
with lesser efficiency on the mental plane. All three levels are subject to the laws of
destiny or karma. But there is also a transcendental part of man that does not abide
by the laws of destiny. "This is the information that Jesus brought to humanity," said
Dora, "a universal model providing human beings with knowledge of universal laws
to guide their existence. Beyond this boundary there is the law of grace. It is due to
this law that prayer makes sense." All course graduates understand the importance of
the law of grace and change their life. Nothing is static: there is always the possibility
of transformation.

The fourth body is the "causal body," the body of happiness, with nine keys. "Intuition always chooses the optimal solution, for the higher good of everyone. There
are various schools that have worked very much on the opening up of the intuitive
plane and cleaning the channels. Geniuses extract their information from this plane:
this is the zone of archetypes. Here is the seed of all things," remarked Dora. Human
beings draw from this level as they evolve and manifest these insights in the physical
plane. The "body of wisdom" is the fifth layer. It is the *vibrational* level at which

wisdom vibrates. No one can give wisdom to someone else, because it is built into us at our birth. Dora remarked that "religions were created at the mental level, but they all contain wisdom." The wisdom from before Creation is intact in all of us, even those who are less wise, but the latter have not made it conscious. "*Life* is the grand master of wisdom!" In Romanian fairy tales, handsome youth usually receives advice from an elderly woman.

The sixth body is "the atmic body," or the superior conscience. "It is your own higher conscience that judges you, not the Divinity," Dora asserted. She spoke of a young woman who died while giving birth to her first child. "Do not be afraid of this moment," Dora said firmly; "it is the most awe-inspiring moment of our life: the eternal life, not the earthly one." The seventh and final body is the "spiritual body." It exists in each and every human being in its complete beauty and perfection. "Here is the kingdom of unconditional love," Dora noted, "the love that doesn't soil, the one that we show towards immaculate beings: a newborn baby, or even the newborn of an animal. It is the pure love; love as principle; the love that lasts and asks for nothing in return." Its source is the seed of light, the spirit, the endless light, placed by divinity at the core of every human.

These seven layers of the human body are like a backpack, filled with everything we need on Earth, the reiki teachers said. The radiant quality of the palms of the human hand is something that all people have at birth. "It was given to us, and it is ours," insisted Dora. Another necessity is the presence of conduits or channels for the distribution of energy: the "subtle channels," known intuitively by our ancestors. "Tradition refers to over 72,000 primary channels of energy, 365,000 when including the secondary ones as well. These channels get clogged, like urban sewerage systems, which get stopped up with refuse. We accumulate refuse and toxins through a poor understanding of alimentation and inadequate breathing. People often become ill because of laziness," Dora said. She referred briefly to the *pranayama* (the art of breathing in Yoga) as a powerful knowledge, now absent in much of the contemporary world. Still, the most toxic things to the human body are negative thoughts and feelings of guilt, resentment, and anger. "No one can heal anyone from the outside. Prescriptions and diets have the role of creating optimal conditions to give the body time to heal itself. A bio-therapist gives energy to stimulate the healing, but healing energy exists in us as the germinative force exists in a wheat grain. The healing energy is within," Dora asserted. That is why someone who is ill should rest in bed for three days, drinking liquids and fasting.

The channels of energy are opened up through a series of tunings, performed by the reiki instructors semi-privately. At the end of the first evening, we were asked into another room one by one and were seated in a chair with our eyes closed while the instructors circled around us quietly, moving their hands in what seemed like circular patterns. I could feel small gusts of air as their palms passed close to my head and body. After a couple of minutes they let me know that I could open my eyes and cheerfully welcomed me "among the Radiants." After the fourth tuning,

Clogged channels

all the participants become "equal at the level of the palms," we were told. When the palms are placed somewhere, energy begins to flow from the center outward. It takes approximately five minutes of laying hands to obtain an effect at the level of the physical body, observable within forty-eight hours. The teachers said that this type of healing is holistic, "pertaining to the whole," and that the medicine of the third millennium will be holistic. Dora and Vlad affirmed that it is not sufficient to make repairs at the level of the physical body: the deeper cause of the illness must be addressed. Nevertheless, the true purpose of Radiant Technique is not healing, but to place the person in direct contact with the source. "We have already entered the Apocalypse," Dora affirmed. Changing the "vibrational nourishment" is necessary at this point. "Time is speeding up," she beckoned. The universal center that exists inside every living thing is characterized by peace and unconditional love. From this center comes the energy that our palms will call to the surface every time it is necessary. Touch is love and the hands are extensions of the heart, Dora added. Both teachers emphasized the inexhaustibility of this power, coming from the Source of Life. They referred to this universal source as the "seed of light," "the spirit," "the endless light." The energy that emanates from this source is called the energy of the heart. This boundless reservoir of divine energy is freely available to all beings, as stated in the biblical verse, "Ask and you shall receive."

Radiant abilities can only be used for good, not for harm, the instructors insisted. Thus, no fear should exist in the heart of the practitioner. Fear is a harmful emotion, they noted. Another crucial guideline for the use of radiant energy is that help should never be denied to anyone or used for material gain. Making a reference to the ethical principles of the New Testament, the teachers insisted that a Real Reiki practitioner should never hesitate to help all who ask for help. They emphasized the need for people to heal each other and themselves on all levels, not just the physical level. The healing force is love, said Dora, and it can never be depleted. When practicing radiant touch, one gives and receives energy equally at the same time. In addition, at the second degree and higher levels, Radiant Technique makes all action possible in the present time: even action directed toward past or future events, or aimed at something or someone at a distance in space. Thus, one can direct energy toward past lives, the moment of conception, the first day of school, the first love, certain moments in the evolution of an illness, the loss of a loved person, a historical or political event, and so on, thus enabling one to become free of energy blockages that could alter present abilities of decision making. The concern with "blockages of energy" was shared by many alternative practitioners I encountered during my fieldwork, expressing a vision of human beings as conduits of life, light, and information.

While engendering an experience of harmony and agency, Real Reiki shares some of the benefits of magical rituals identified by Bronislaw Malinowski (1992 [1948]): alleviating anxiety about uncontrollable, distant, or unknown events by focusing the mind and the body on a precise sequence of signs, sensations, symbols, and actions. Because functionalist explanations of ritual privileged the system over individuals, they obscured the fact that the observer's own rationality was also a cultural product, denying full agency and instrumentality to participants. From a person-centered anthropological perspective, rituals and magic are forms of agency embedded in the local cultural matrix of relationships and emotions as well as meaningful ways of knowing and relating. While providing ways to perpetuate society and negotiate contradictions, magical practices represent a space for engagement with possibilities and alternatives, personal, mythical, or social. Students of Radiant Technique get in touch, literally and figuratively, with new sites of personal power and meaning, acquiring another means to connect to others physically, spiritually, and emotionally. In the process of becoming "Radiants," participants become enfranchised and learn to experience enhanced selves, as conduits of the universe's creative forces and agents of healing, capable to give energy to oneself and others, or influence distant persons or events in time and space. From level three one becomes "a conscious co-creator with the Divinity," in the teachers' enthusiastic words.

The instructors said that avenues of reception of universal energy are nine-fold:

1. sun exposure, in a gradual manner, as people have receptors of vital energy all over their bodies (identified with *prana* in Yoga).
2. breathing, as in the nasal *fossae* there are more receptors of energy; this offers the greatest percentage of absorption; pine forests and waterfalls are richest.
3. consumption of liquids, especially water, having the greatest capacity to store vital energy; in second place: crystals; best: water energized in green bottles.
4. consumption of "living food": uncooked vegetables, legumes, fruit, and grains.
5. Radiant Technique: feeding the other seven bodies integrally through Real Reiki energization and harmonization.
6. sleep, as some of the bodies leave and acquire information from other sources.
7. practicing positive thinking and good deeds, based on the principle of resonance: "law of the boomerang: what goes out also comes back."
8. walks or strolls, as we intersect energy fields that cover the entire earth.
9. songs, which exert two forms of influence: passive (when we listen to music) and active (when we sing, even if we sing out of tune). "Try to sing and think negatively: it is not possible," affirmed Dora; "it raises the level of the vibrations." The central reservoir of these vibrations is the solar plexus. Stress depletes it.

The energy of this reservoir is distributed along the seven energy centers along the spine. The teachers drew a sketch of the human spine and drew seven spots along its length, from one near the coccyx (tailbone) to seven above the skull. The energy center near the coccyx is the *chakra muladhara*; to bring it to resonance one can use acoustic vibrations, such as the musical note C, or light vibrations in the color red. The second energy center is near the umbilicus (bellybutton), two inches below: the *hara* center in martial arts and also the *chakra svadisthana*. The musical note D or the color orange can be used to energize it. The plexus (chest) is associated with the third energy center, *chakra manipura,* energized by the note E and the yellow light. The fourth center is near the heart, *chakra anahata*, and associated with the note F and the color green, "the color of healing." The thyroid gland (base of the neck) is the site for *chakra vishudhi*, which can be energized by the musical note G and the color blue. The sixth, *chakra ajna*, is also "the third eye," in the middle of the forehead, energized by the note A and the color indigo. Finally atop the head is *chakra sahashrara*, associated with the musical note B and vibrating to the color violet (purple).

Dora and Vlad went on to draw the shape of a human palm, stating that each of the energy centers and the vital organs previously described had projections all over the surface of the body, on the chest, on the iris of the eye, on the surface of the tongue, on the ear, soles of the feet, and palms of the hand. For example, the coccyx corresponds to the center point on the inside of the wrist, the umbilicus to the tip of the thumb, the thyroid to the index finger ("the finger of light" said Dora), the plexus to the middle finger, the third eye to the ring finger, the heart to the tip of the pinky, and the top of the head to the center of the palm. The teachers recalled a traditional Christian practice of putting the palm on top of one's head and reciting the Lord's Prayer: "this brings into resonance all the seven energy centers." Another mythological connection: the sixth center (the third eye) projects on the heel of the foot, "thus the legend of Achilles' heel."

A session of holistic energization and optimization consists of three sets of four positions of the hands on the body. "It is not a treatment," the teachers insisted. The first set of four positions takes twenty minutes as follows: the palms are placed over the eyes for five minutes, over the temples for five minutes, over the back of the neck for five minutes, and over the front of the neck for five more minutes. This can be done in the morning. In the afternoon, another twenty-minute sequence should be performed: five minutes on the chest, five on the plexus (lower chest/under the breasts), five minutes on the belly, palms laid on both sides of the bellybutton, and five minutes on the lower belly, near the fold of the thighs. The last set of energizing positions can be practiced in the evening: on the top of the back for five minutes (the trapeze muscles), underneath the back plates (on the lower back ribs) for five minutes, on the kidneys for five minutes, and on the coccyx for the final five minutes. An ill person can benefit greatly from a "Circle of Radiants" laying hands on him or her: the more radiants participate, the more doses of energization the patient can receive during a given time. The sequence of these positions is important, remarked Dora and Vlad, but one may take a break between positions if one wishes. All twelve hand positions have to be performed in the prescribed sequence for the energy and harmony of the whole to be restored.

Three homework assignments were given after the first night: to carry out a complete session of energization, to keep a record of all the instances in which the hands touch different objects within the first fifteen minutes after waking the next morning, and to bring a crystal to energize on the next (final) day of the course. Before departing, the teachers shared two more applications: the first was the greeting *Shanti* ("peace" in Sanskrit), a way of honoring someone or something, accompanied by union of the palms in front of the chest; the second was the "hug": yes, the all-American hug, praised by the instructors as a highly desirable healing touch practice.

The following morning we were greeted with "Welcome among Radiants!" and taught various frequencies and applications for holistic energization and optimization on others: people, animals, plants (houseplants as well as fruit trees or trees in the forest), minerals, as well as for those who are mildly ill or gravely ill. Participants were informed of three golden rules: (1) never offer your services or help to people who have not asked for it; (2) do not refuse anyone who has asked for your help, even if it is 2:00 A.M.; and (3) never offer your services with an ulterior motive, hoping to gain something.

Dora suggested another exercise for the two weeks following the reiki course: "Everything you touch, do it with a gracefulness as if the entire physical body participates in a cosmic dance; be a caress; the energy of love flows constantly through the palms, but if it is made conscious it is richer. Thus you can attract others, by being open channels and indeed Radiants! Wherever it passes, that which is alive leaves its cosmic print. The *etheric* aura of the earth contains these prints." She spoke of hope, trust, and positive thinking as heritage. The energy of love can be put in food and in all gestures and words. "If you approach someone with love, you are already helping them heal. Caress the doorknob, even at work. You reap what you sow, except tenfold," Dora said.

The teachers recommended that a full energizing session of the twelve positions should be carried out every few days, to restore the energy of the whole. The processes of life consume energy, which should normally be replenished through sleep. They described sleep as "a secondary pilot, like a cleaning lady who cleans up and evacuates refuse; the physical body is cleansed by the subconscious; the soul travels towards the primordial source: our spiritual masters." People ought to wake up rested and in good spirits, she said, "otherwise it means that the soul has remained in inferior zones." Every person has his or her own deposit of energy. Central deposits are the heart for joy or happiness, the liver for sorrow or sadness, and the kidneys for argument or conflict. "Remember," Dora admonished: "I make my problems, I decide my life. Try to be the master of your own ship." The teachers warned that three weeks after beginning these energizing practices, it is possible for symptoms of old diseases to reappear, a "crisis of healing," common to natural therapies. Also, the tunings can cause sleepiness for several days.

During the "second degree" course, Dora and Vlad suggested a "fast of silence." Much like a food fast, it enables a "coupling" with one's inner center—the place where peace, harmony, and "the absolute" reside. Fasting can bring about cleansing and connectedness, the key to its fruitfulness being regular practice. "Our servants make noise," Dora said, referring to our physical and emotional bodies. The mind is especially loud and distracting with its relentless plans, regrets, and guilt. The voice of the divine is often difficult to hear over the racket, but the inner guide never abandons anyone. Light and God are delicate and considerate, Dora said; "they do not penetrate our hearts and lives if we do not invite them in." The teachers went on to speak about the Word as a sacrament (*taină*) and a creator. It became embodied and became human for us humans. Our words are "co-creators": we co-create through utterance and speak through breath. They asserted that every word launched into the world is "alive" and molds the world. "Your word should be like a caress," Dora prompted. The fast of silence rests the neck chakra, giving one's words additional healing power and enables energetic recharging.

A most important aspect of words is "force," the teachers noted. Loving words must be also uttered with force and require courage. Light is more powerful than darkness, and we are made of light. Words uttered take root and yield results. Therefore, the first word spoken after leaving the fast of silence is very important. The teachers spoke of the "superior planes of existence"—the realm of the Holy Trinity—and advised second degree initiates regarding the recitation of the Lord's prayer. They pointed out that the line "hallowed be thy name" is addressed to the Father; "thy kingdom come" refers to Christ; and "thy will be done," to the work of the Spirit. They recommended a pause before saying "give us this day our daily bread," which allows the person praying to stay in touch with the "Superior Divine Trinity" a little longer. "Then, you may continue with the lower realms: the requests, etc.," they conceded.

For several months after the course, I regularly practiced on myself the twelve hand positions aimed at restoring the energy of the whole being. I did this at night, before falling sleep, and sometimes during the day. These quiet sessions were exercises in patience, relaxation, and imagination, "experimental" leaps that charged my body with universal energy. I have not persisted in that kind of self-care, but the experience did influence my awareness and appreciation of the connective and communicative potential of "laying hands," touching, or the simple gesture of holding the hands *over* something.

The Real Reiki method was deftly contextualized within the spiritual and social worlds of the participants, drawing on Orthodox symbols, narratives, and traditions, while forging links between traditional Romanian spirituality and the language of Radiance, with which it resonates on a various levels. The divine healing energy that constitutes the basis of this practice is referred to as the "energy of the heart" (*energia inimii*), a description that resonates with the Orthodox monastic practice called the Prayer of the Heart (*rugăciunea inimii*) or Jesus Prayer, central to Hesychasm. Radiant Technique postulates a permeable yet powerful body–mind, which can be engaged actively and creatively in transforming one's condition and the conditions of others, past or future. Reiki discourse rejects the materialist objectification of human beings, portraying persons as conscious vessels of divine energy and co-creators of the universe rather than mere victims of disease, historical circumstances, or economic and political inequities. In Dora's words, there is "a transcendental part of man that does not abide by the laws of destiny." Human beings are able to cultivate their virtues while helping others, to take an active and conscious role in their own well-being, and to seek to transform themselves for the purpose of achieving a different state of health, happiness, or wisdom. Radiant Technique challenges linear and mechanistic conceptions of space and time as well as the notion of the person as bounded and ruled by self-interest, characteristic of Western modernity. In fact, Radiant Technique postulates and supports a relational view of personhood and a sense of connectedness with the natural world and human others. The discourse of radiance also rejects pervasive cost–benefit calculations of market capitalism as it centers on the notion that the most significant universal resource is a natural and inherent quality of all living things, a power accessible from within the body, free of charge, in endless supply.

Ascent into the Future: Aromatherapy, Art, and Science, Ancient and Modern

Long before becoming one of the most popular forms of alternative therapy in the United Kingdom's National Health Service, the use of aromatic plant extracts and essences played an important role in all great medical traditions. As far back as ancient Egypt, 5,000 years ago, cedarwood oil served for embalming and hygiene. In India and China fragrant oils were widely used several millennia before the classical Greek ancestor of modern medicine Hippocrates (500 B.C.E.) advised on aromatic baths and scented massage every day, or Christian scriptures encoded the use of almost two hundred plant oils (Williams 2004:5). Price and Price (1999) note that modern methods of distillation resemble closely the methods used by early Chinese and Islamic scientists to produce oils, having remained much the same for millennia. Yet aromatherapy by its current name is a mid-twentieth-century creation, being a subset of phytotherapy, the treatment with medicinal plants. More recently, aromatology is being used as a more inclusive label, which includes internal use of aromatic oils, particularly by French practitioners.

Aromatherapy uses numerous common herbs and spices that are popular in diverse culinary traditions and originate in various structural components of plants, including basil, celery, chamomile, clove, ginger, lemon, oregano, peppermint, rosemary, tarragon, thyme, and turmeric. All of these have a dazzling array of medicinal properties, including anti-inflammatory, anti-spasmodic, digestive stimulant, or anxiolytic (relieving anxiety). In contrast to the magic-bullet model of biomedicine, aromatic plants have a multitude of effects and may benefit a variety of conditions. This has been documented in many traditional societies, where nearby cultural groups may use the same plant in different ways, for different purposes, or use different parts of the plant. Furthermore, the same plant or oil may have apparently contradictory effects that practitioners describe as "balancing" or *adaptogenic*: acting as a stimulant on some occasions and as a sedative on others, raising blood pressure in one case but lowering it in another (Price and Price 1999:76). Citrus oils aid in digestion, while also being invaluable as deodorants: it is widely agreed that they effectively neutralize many odors, rather than mask them, and are becoming valuable in creating a pleasant ambiance in burn units and other healing situations when bad smells are generated, such as incontinence, that have a negative impact on the mood of patients and caregivers alike (Price and Price 1999:76).

An important property common among many essential oils is their antibacterial action: some species of thyme kill staphylococcus and are being used to create Earth-friendly and nontoxic household disinfectants. Another oil testifying to the complex and powerful chemistry of traditional plant oils is pungent neem oil. It is popular in Ayurvedic medicine as a carrier oil and skin rash remedy, and contains more than forty distinct *limonoids*, fatty acids, glycerides, and sulfur compounds. Limonoids are aromatic plant chemicals with diverse healing properties, including antibacterial, antiviral, antifungal, antimalarial, antioxidant, antimutagenic, antineoplastic (anti-cancer), anti-proliferative, antihemorrhagic, antidiarrheal, antisecretory, antiulcer, antihyperglycaemic, and immunomodulatory. In an article on the medicinal properties of neem leaves, Indian biochemists Subapriya and Nagini (2005) note that over 140 compounds were found in neem and that medicinal uses exist for every part of the plant: "leaves, flowers, seeds, fruits, roots and bark."

G. Brahmachari (2004) of Natural Product Laboratory in Santiniketan, West Bengal, calls neem "an omnipotent plant" and a "wonder tree." Neem has a prominent role in the indigenous medicines of the Indian subcontinent, treating ailments from diarrhea to tumors. Neem extracts have also been used as insecticides in traditional farming, to spray on plants and seeds. Southeast Asian and African scientists searching for ways to prevent malaria infection anticipate that using neem to control mosquito larvae may be a cost-effective and sustainable strategy. The work of Indian biochemists from Tamil Nadu is at the forefront of new drug research exploring medical applications of traditional plants such as neem in modern laboratories: certain limonoids from the neem tree (*Azadirachta indica*) have anticancer properties, inducing apoptosis (self-destruction) in cancer cells (Priyadarsini et al. 2010; Harish et al. 2010). Traditionally a remedy for diarrhea, neem has been demonstrated effective against multidrug-resistant *Vibrio cholerae* in a laboratory setting (Thakurta et al. 2007). In testing a patented neem extract, German zoologists (Schmahl et al. 2010) found that "a broad range of pests and parasites," from house dust mites to bed bugs could be controlled with the neem extract mixed with shampoo or water. Dutch entomologists (Boeke et al. 2004) concluded that some toxicity can occur with chronic ingestion of neem-based pesticide residues (reproductive effects in mammals), but if used carefully, neem products can be safe. Most toxic effects appear to be reversible.

Aromatherapist, pharmacist, and founder of the California company Aroma Rx, Inc., Michelle Williams (2004) begins her book *Only the Essentials* with the legal disclaimer that "healing and medicine are two distinct fields," and that its content should not be substituted for the advice of a health professional. The paradoxical

[handwritten margin note: Old medicine rejected by Western Medicine]

and contested status of ancient healing practices in the legalistic arena of biomedical health care is vividly expressed. Substances like neem that have been in use for thousands of years are an embodiment of this paradox: as alternative medicines, they are coming under new scrutiny, some being restricted and labeled "poison," for public safety. It is ironic that one can have the freedom to test unproven drugs on oneself in clinical trials or work as a professional guinea pig, rights granted by democratic state governments, but not the authority to distribute or sell traditional products for consumption or therapeutic purposes. The latter is increasingly restricted in Western countries, where the politics of health and food production have led to branding herbal therapies as "untested," a status below placebos, palliatives, or risky alternatives.

[handwritten margin note: Proper Amounts]

While agreeing that essential oils can be hazardous and should be labeled as such, aromatherapists Len and Shirley Price remark in the tradition of Paracelsus that many (if not most) substances can cause harm if used improperly, for example, underripe potatoes, excess alcohol, or too much aspirin (Price and Price 1999:55–6). But while many of us have recent local and collective experiences to guide us in the use of potatoes, fermented beverages, or over-the-counter analgesics, urbanized Westerners have grown increasingly unfamiliar with (and unable to rely on) traditional knowledge of aromatic substances, or their own interpretation of sensory impressions, particularly when it comes to benefits, uses, and efficacy of scented plants. This creates a new and growing need for persons with official expertise in aromatherapy and phytotherapy. Aromatherapy is becoming professionalized and incorporated into patient care, especially in areas of hospice and palliative care. It is also being used in working with young people who have developmental and learning difficulties, sufferers of anxiety and depression, and persons with chronic stress, often in combination with massage therapy and other holistic methods of promoting well-being, such as music.

In the foreword to *Only the Essentials*, titled "About the Author," Michelle Williams describes her mission as one of empowerment: to allow consumers to be "their own health advocates." Simultaneously, she cautions of the dangers of self-reliance: highly concentrated, some plant oils can be irritating to the skin, making it prone to sunburn, other oils may produce liver toxicity, and yet others can have carcinogenic or hormonal effects; many of these are prohibited or restricted by the International Fragrance Association (IFRA). Echoing a classic cultural adage that humans need to be wary of untamed natural forces, Williams (2004:21) warns that "natural" does not equal "safe," cautioning consumers against various risks, including certain oils that may have negative consequences for particular persons. Pregnant women, asthmatics, and cancer patients are more vulnerable to adverse effects. Due to their small size and sensitive skin, children need highly diluted oils (1 percent instead of 2 percent).

Williams (2004) popularizes aromatherapy by blending scientific terminology with the language of sensations, self-care, and eco-consciousness. While speaking of plant oils and their sweet, fresh, clean, or musky smells, abundantly embodied in their origins and mode of action, she also speaks of spirit, vitality, and global transformation. Williams describes essential oils as agents of plants' therapeutic powers, vehicles of vitamins and phytohormones that penetrate through skin and olfactory nerves into the nose and brain. Scientists do not have a definitive explanation of how aromatherapy works, she writes, but our sense of smell is 10,000 times more sensitive than that of taste. Humans can process up to 100,000 different smells, which can regulate moods, behaviors, and sexual desire while reducing stress-related discomforts (Williams 2004:16). Concentrated and volatile, oils may be extracted from various parts of the plant: "flower, leaf, blossom petal, resin, tree, bark, root, twig, seed, berry, bark and rhizome," and they tend to be sensitive to heat and light. Echoing the sentiments of Native American shamans, Williams describes these oils as "the soul of the plant," an expression of a "quintessential" life force or vital essence (Williams 2004:3). Many factors influence the quality and effectiveness of an essential oil: the plant variety and the amount of plant used, the part of the plant, and the place and time of harvest, including the time of the day, soil quality, climate, and weather.

From being a classical healing art, aromatherapy is now becoming a global industry. There is increasing competition for authority and for the buying power and loyalty of consumers, who seek "value" or bargains and lack the necessary background to choose the best product on the market. In contemporary societies, brand names (rather than the apothecary's reputation) provide assurance regarding the reliable composition and efficacy of herbal products. An alarmist tone rings among certain aromatherapists regarding industrial-scale commercialization and practices of standardization, as well as the use of synthetic oils, on the grounds of their unique and complex status as natural essences. In their comprehensive volume *Aromatherapy for Health Professionals*, aromatherapists Shirley and Len Price (1999:25) write that "it is important to preserve the wholeness of an essential oil in order to guard its natural synergy (from the Greek *syn* = together, *ergon* = work)," and any alteration may upset the balance of the elements in the oil. Ingredients do not work separately but together, in concert. They note that in the wild many plants, such as thyme, appear as different chemotypes, each yielding a distinct oil "in makeup and therapeutic action" and that different subtypes of lavender yield oils that have "different properties and indications"—yet such different plants or oils may be lumped together in the British Pharmacopoeia (BP) products stocked in hospital pharmacies, along with incomplete or even synthetic oils, making them unreliable for use in aromatherapy. While standardization is touted as a central goal of biomedicine and the pharmaceutical industry, and lack thereof is voiced by skeptics as a common criticism of natural supplements and CAM products, practices of standardizing essential oils to produce the same thing each time contradict the local and contingent nature of how plants grow in their natural environments and their embeddedness in local soils, environments, and economies. Unlike things manufactured in laboratories under highly controlled conditions, plants do not always grow the same or produce identical blends of compounds in the same proportions. This natural diversity is difficult to manage in a biomedical setting, where products and procedures are constantly being streamlined and there is overwhelming preference for cheaper generics and budget-minded alternatives.

This perspective on the healing power of the essential oils is in vivid contrast to the approaches of biomedical scientists cited earlier, who examine distinct ingredients in isolation (such as the compound *azadirachtin* in neem), in a laboratory setting, trying to identify and quantify the exact biochemical and molecular mechanisms involved and which amounts produce specific biological effects. In the eyes of holistically minded aromatherapists, the power of the essential oil for aromatherapy purposes is significantly undermined by attempts to "divide and conquer" scientifically, echoing the language of philosophical and religious traditions that equated wholeness and holiness.

Current Practice: Medical Aromatherapy

The growing litigiousness of developed societies and the fact that the complexity of herbal medicines and their variability makes it difficult to test their effects and risks in clinical trials have contributed to a lot of hesitancy from orthodox medical practitioners and politicians who perceive traditional remedies as unproven, despite an ample history of successful use and effectiveness. Nevertheless, Price and Price (1999:62) note that surveys from the United Kingdom and Israel showed that 60–90 percent of physicians had referred their patients to alternative health practitioners, whereas in Canada and the United States, more than 70 percent would like to learn more about the therapies available. Aromatherapy has achieved some of its widest acceptance in the United Kingdom, where it is increasingly integrated into biomedical settings, particularly through nursing care.

Many UK hospitals are funding nurses' aromatherapy courses. As Price and Price echo the biomedical discourse that demands for practitioners to have "precise control" over substances used, they insist that there are very few side effects documented compared to allopathic medicines, such as antibiotics, that essential oils are nonpolluting to the environment (unlike synthetic substances), and that they tend to have multiple benefits, unlike pharmaceutical drugs; they describe essential oil molecules as pro- and eu-biotic, rather than anti-biotic, being aggressive to germs but harmless to humans (Price and Price 1999:64–65). They explain that the reason plant oils can correct deficits or blockages is that biochemically, essential oils have much in common with steroids and proteins in the human body (steroids such as cholesterol, vitamin D, or cortisone and amino acids, the building blocks of proteins), agents for energy transformation. Thus, we come full circle to the notion of the sun and its energy as the fundamental agents of healing: "plants capture electromagnetic energy from the sun and some of this is stored in the essential oil" (Price and Price 1999:78).

As fundamentally "natural" as plant oils may be, when used for aromatherapy in the United Kingdom they have the legal status of medicines and both their prescription and application must follow legal and institutional protocols. A new ruling will significantly restrict the distribution of many popular plant-based products in the name of consumer safety, creating controversy, since it appears to discriminate against smaller producers and suppliers. In France, a law was voted on in 1990 and applied for several years that forbade reimbursement for plant medicines, including essential oils. As of 2010, plant-based medicines are considered supplements in the United States. Not being regulated by the Food and Drug Administration (thus not subjected to clinical testing and standardization), they are not reimbursable by insurance or eligible for tax-sheltered spending. Periodically, government authorities move to gain greater control over the production and circulation of plant-based therapeutics by instituting new (often costly) procedures, norms, and fees.

In her detailed work *Clinical Aromatherapy*, practicing nurse and academic researcher Jane Buckle (2003:130–1) recommends a variety of ways in which aromatherapy can be used in hospitals, with a gentle touch, such as the "m" technique, a technique "simple enough for a 5-year old child to do," that can involve family, a technique that is "empowering for the giver and beneficial for the receiver" (Buckle 2003:154). This is a registered method of touch therapy that uses constant light pressure and a prescribed sequence of moves, each repeated three times, in a set pattern; this approach is supposed to instill confidence and has a strong calming, almost hypnotic, effect on fragile and troubled patients, who often fall asleep afterwards (Buckle 2003:152–3). The "m" technique is gaining popularity in U.S. hospitals, being used in a New York City hospital to relax patients prior to surgery. Whereas in the United States, laws governing the use of CAM vary state by state, approximately half of U.S. states allow nurses to use a range of healing resources, but nurses are expected to meet the standard of the "highest" or most rigorous credential that the nurse holds (Buckle 2003:395–7). Despite the ample evidence available on the efficacy of essential oils for many discomforts, some of the websites of hospital-based alternative medicine guides in the United States affirm that all effects of essential oils besides the mood modulating effects are scientifically unproven (aspencancerguide. org 2011). Jane Buckle notes that in the climate of worker shortage and overwork that currently characterizes the nursing profession in the United States, these methods provide additional empowerment and caring for patients while bringing tremendous stress relief to staff and patients alike.

While scientific evidence behind aromatherapy is growing and its relative status is becoming re-labeled as "complementary" to orthodox medical care, practitioners are challenged to balance science with art. As with other alternative and complementary practices, the professionalization phenomenon entails acceptance and incorporation into the mainstream of health care. With that comes the increased financial security of reimbursement by insurers or national health systems along with a constant submission to oversight, judgments, and limitations based on biomedical and institutional models of efficacy. Often the acceptance of secondary status is required as well, such as designation as supportive or adjuvant therapy. Licensing and regulation limits access to the profession and high-status ranks of official therapists by instituting the demand that practitioners understand the chemistry of their *material medica*, not only

Cont'

the properties, effects, and interactions of the essential oils. In the United Kingdom, practitioners can obtain training and expertise as well as liability insurance. They are also accountable legally and professionally and are expected to follow criteria for practice and standards for the administration of medicines, including authorization by supervisors, consultation with other medical practitioners on a team, consent of patient or legal guardian, documentation of the care plan, and evaluation of effectiveness, which must be noted in the patient's record (Price and Price 1999:272).

Some practitioners hope that the use of aromatherapy in nursing may foster a revival of the art of nursing care (Price and Price 1999:261). The ability of essential oils to regulate moods, promote relaxation, and induce sleep, among the other benefits they may provide, represents a valuable resource for modern health care, not only by reducing the need for addictive sedatives and tranquilizers that may interact with other medicines but also by providing delight, stimulation, and comfort to patients and their often harried caregivers. As the relationship between caregivers and patients has been much abbreviated, depersonalized, and automated as a result of technological advancements, budgetary constraints, and the capitalist organization of work and illness (in which people are rarely cared for by those who are familiar to them), medical aromatherapy is an opportunity to tap the power of our sensoria as doorways to other modes of experience and relationality. Our noses, our skins, and our minds are thus awakened from patient passivity to engage us in the process of living through illness, even if overcoming it is an improbable goal.

Polythetic Medicine

Scheper-Hughes and Lock (1987:10) have noted that "we lack a precise vocabulary with which to deal with mind-body-society interactions and so we are left suspended in hyphens, testifying to the disconnectedness of our thoughts." Various fragmented and hybrid concepts attempt to bridge the analytic and conceptual fractures (biosocial, mind-body, psychosomatic), including the popular concept of CAM, a mouthful that has been reduced to a syllable that sounds disturbingly similar to scam, and implicitly positions these numerous and diverse practices in a minefield of questionable authority and potential risk. Thus I suggest the need for a new term that dispenses with the fractured, hegemonic, and administrative flavor and baggage that is captured in the term "CAM," alternative medicine, or unorthodox medicine. The notion of integrative medicine is much more appealing, and it seems quite appropriate to the current trend of medical syncretism, but it also echoes bits and pieces of colonial, imperialistic, and modernistic ethos of incorporation, in the suggestion that it is a blended solution. Just as marginal yet bountiful lands, resources, and subjects were slated for integration into the empire and developed, often to their oblivion, the "other" medicines are currently on schedule to be integrated, domesticated, sanitized, deodorized, measured, standardized, professionalized, and perhaps made to smell and taste like nothing alien at all.

Undoubtedly, integrative medicine may be better Western medicine for the twenty-first century, but it is unlikely to capture or reproduce the richness and complexity or the range of efficacy of the incorporated medical traditions and their practitioners. For the continuation and development of the non-Western medical traditions on their own terms, diverse shamanic traditions, spirit-healing traditions, indigenous and folk healing traditions, and the manifold creative blends of these mind-body-society therapies, I urge the creation of a new cultural category, one that can sit lightly among other taxonomic entities as an umbrella term for all of these "alternative practices" that may not be amenable to integration or complementarity, yet valuable, meaningful, supportive and efficacious when assessed on their own terms, rather than by standards of biomedical science or political and economic considerations. The gloss of *polythetic* medicine would describe these practices and practitioners better than terms currently in use by being inclusive, yet less hegemonic. The term was introduced to social anthropology by Rodney Needham (1975) in his article, "Polythetic Classification: Convergence and Consequences," published thirty-six years ago in *Man* and preceded by the following abstract:

The conventional definition of a conceptual class is that its members must possess certain properties in common. Vygotsky and Wittgenstein have shown that this definition is unrealistic and logically unnecessary. The resultant recognition of classificatory concepts formed by family resemblances has recently led to a revision of anthropological analyses of kinship and of belief statements. The present article reports the discovery that, by a remarkable convergence of ideas in the past decade, family resemblance predicates had already been adduced in certain natural sciences under the term "polythetic classification." The methodological and experimental results of this approach are set out, and a variety of consequences for social anthropology are drawn from them. A main conclusion is that comparative studies carried out in the stock classificatory terms of anthropology are subverted by the realization that they refer not to common features but to polythetic classes of social facts. It is suggested that effective comparison may nevertheless be practicable by reliance on a purely formal terminology of analytical concepts, and it is envisaged that these may permit the determination of basic predicates in the study of human affairs.

Another possibility would be going beyond the orthodox/unorthodox polarity with a term such as *heterodox* medicine. A drawback of both of the above terms could be their Greek origin, which grounds the taxonomic practice of labeling these traditions with one word as a classificatory practice squarely in the naturalistic genealogy to Western methods and habits of knowledge making, and still masks the manifold origins, foundations, and experiential complexities of these practices. It seems that an older Sanskrit term might be more politically correct, maybe *atman* medicine, for example, since *atman* refers to the soul, real self, or "true self." But the most correct would likely be a word that means self or spirit in one of the endangered native languages of small-scale societies in Africa, the Pacific Islands, or the Americas, whose cultures and identities are being globalized and whose traditional knowledge is being blended into the giant cauldron of global progress. Not surprisingly,

[margin: There are different definitions of power]

[margin: Who now Anecdotal has value too]

skeptics, critics, and debunkers of CAM have argued that there is only one kind of medicine, medicine that has been *proven* to work. They contend that once an alternative medical practice is proven safe and effective by scientific standards, it ceases to be alternative: it is just medicine.

A number of anthropologists, sociologists, and historians of "unorthodox" medicine and non-Western healing traditions have drawn on the scholarship of Thomas Kuhn (1996 [1962]), whose influential book *The Structure of Scientific Revolutions* adopted the Greek word *paradigm,* meaning pattern or example, to describe dominant scientific theories that capture the imagination of entire cultures or generations of scientists and remain unchallenged by data for long periods of time, during which scientists work fervently to build up supportive data and cumulative insights, in a process Kuhn described as "normal science." In contrast, revolutionary science takes place when enough exceptions to the old paradigm accumulate to trigger the dissolution or substantial revision of the previous theory or paradigm. It is definitely the case that the absolute dominance of "orthodox" medicine and its particular brand of mind-body dualism is on the wane and that thousands of researchers all over the world (including in China, India, Europe, and North America) are producing studies that investigate the effectiveness of CAM therapies, with promising results.

A quick Internet search in PubMed, Medscape, or Science Direct reveals that the number of studies on complementary and alternative medicine has skyrocketed over the past ten years. Thus, the paradigm of mechanistic-body-medicine has begun to be supplanted by the paradigm of CAM and a desire by health professionals and institutions to incorporate CAM into their existing bag of tricks. This adoption of CAM into the world of biomedicine is certainly, at least in part, a wise business move, sprung from the desire to satisfy customers and offer a wider range of services and products. The increasing involvement of health professionals in CAM has generated a proliferation of programs, certificates, and integrative health centers, along with a plethora of small businesses that provide wellness enhancement through massage, nutritional counseling, relaxation, tai chi, and yoga. Mainstream medical practitioners and administrative officials continue to call for regulation and licensure, which threatens small producers of remedies and traditional practitioners without clinical medical degrees, whose expertise is based on experiential learning, such as apprenticeship, whose credibility relies mainly on reputation, and who tend to lack the resources to compete with clinical providers for clients or challenge regulatory restrictions. Since the 1990s there has been a rapidly growing recognition of the fact that a great number of people have a need and a desire to be treated holistically, that there is a mental-emotional-spiritual-social dimensionality to illness, and that attending to these complexities as a matter of course can improve clinical outcomes and the caregiving relationship, as well as increase the satisfaction of providers, particularly in cases when there is chronic or incurable illness, while there is still the possibility of enhancing a patient's well-being through palliative care.

QUESTIONS FOR CLASS DISCUSSION

1. What are some of your earliest or strongest memories of pleasant sensations? Do you think that they were shaped or mediated by cultural factors? How about biological ones?
2. If you were to choose one way of moving for the next ten minutes that would provide you with an extremely positive and refreshing experience, what would it be and why?
3. Think about five reasons why you may experience reluctance about touching an old person. What would make it easier and more pleasant for both of you?

QUESTIONS FOR ESSAY WRITING

1. Describe a place, person, or event that you remember because of the smell(s), whether pleasant or unpleasant, and reflect on the relationship between smell and well-being.
2. Choose a color and research its significance in a particular culture, comparing it with the uses and meanings of that color in your culture and your own life experience.
3. Think of some of your oldest favorite songs, experiences, or memories involving sound(s). How do they make you feel? What other memories, emotions, or sensations do you elicit by singing or revisiting them in your thoughts. Do these surprise you? Why?
4. Explore a distinctive or repetitive sound that is commonly encountered in your culture in one of these environments: school, hospital, nursing home, grocery store, restaurant, kitchen, gym, street, beach, and so on. What thoughts, ideas, or feelings does it elicit in you?
5. Describe your favorite movement experience. How about your second favorite? Third?

SUGGESTED READINGS

Classen, Constance (ed.) (2005), *The Book of Touch (Sensory Formations)*. Oxford: Berg.

Classen, Constance, David Howes, and Anthony Synnott (eds.) (1994), *Aroma: The Cultural History of Smell*. New York: Routledge

Howes, David (ed.) (2009), *The Sixth Sense Reader (Sensory Formations)*. Oxford: Berg.

Hughes, Kerry, M.Sc. (2007), *The Incense Bible: Plant Scents That Transcend World Culture, Medicine, and Spirituality*. Binghamton, NY: The Haworth Press.

Schnaubelt, Kurt (1999), *Medical Aromatherapy: Healing with Essential Oils*. Berkeley, CA: Frog, Ltd.

RECOMMENDED FILMS

Complementary Health Therapies in England (1992), *Aromatherapy in a Cardiac Surgery Ward* (31 min); Complementary Health Therapies in England (1992), *Touching: Reflexology and Massage for AIDS* (87 min); both films by Philip Singer, Health Behavioral Sciences Program, Oakland University, School of Health Sciences, Rochester, MI 48309 (313/370–4038)

Eat Drink Man Woman (1994), dir. Ang Lee; an aging chef and his three daughters.

Like Water for Chocolate (1992), dir. Alfonso Arau; screenplay by Laura Esquivel, based on her award-winning novel, published in 1990; love, cooking, and magical elements.

Scent of a Woman (1992), dir. Martin Brest; a youth accompanies a spirited blind man.

Shall We Dance? (1996), dir. Masayuki Suo; accountant finds passion in dance lessons.

INTERNET RESOURCES

Dr. Hugo Heyrman / Belgian Synesthesia Association: http://www.doctorhugo.org/synaesthesia/.
National Association of Creative Arts Therapies Associations: http://www.nccata.org/index.htm.
Sensory Studies: http://www.sensorystudies.org/.
Tai chi–related medical research articles from Tree of Life Tai Chi in Boston: http://www.treeoflifetaichi.com/medicalresearch.html.
TRI (2011) Touch Research Institute at the University of Miami Medical School: http://www6.miami.edu/touch-research/InfantMassage.html.

–5–

Conclusion: Looking into the Future of Alternative Medicine

An orthodox attempt at concluding would provide a brief assessment of the state of affairs and make a reasoned prediction about the future of alternative medicine. From a postmodern, post-pasteurian, and post-rationalist perspective, however, I feel compelled to concur with Emily Martin's finale to her analysis of immunity and flexibility in American culture, a reflection "on the impossibility of concluding":

> In part, it is impossible to conclude because there is no vantage point from which I can say confidently that the developments that I have described are "good" or "bad." Or, rather, there is no *one* vantage point but instead a very great *many* vantage points from which such evaluations can be made. In a sense, the structure of the book itself, tracking its way from one vantage point to another but making none of them the foundation, is an index of this feature of the world we are making. (1994:249)

Because of the polythetic and fluctuating nature of alternative medicine, a similar disclaimer is surely in order. I recognize the structure of the book to be an act of *bricolage* or *pastiche*, to borrow the texture and nuance of French cultural critique: it is a quilt of voices, arguments, histories, interpretations, and sensualities that reflects the contribution of numerous people, extremely diverse traditions, and just as numerous cross-pollinations in the arena of health, illness, and healing. The contemporary world of alternative medicine and CAM is a complex system, characterized by vibrancy, flux, and the impossibility of fully controlling or predicting where it will end. There is a feeling of "empowered powerlessness" when one attempts to understand health as being simultaneously and perhaps equally a personal, local, and global issue, one that is entangled with politics, science, religions, communities, relationships, environmental challenges, and everyday choices.

As Martin aptly wrote: "We are not victims of a sinister plot perpetuated by villainous others, but active participants in a complex process" (1994:249). I am compelled to expand on her optimistic statement however, to add that some people in our world (including this writer) can easily become at various times "victims," not of plots, but of structural violence, inequalities, intimidation, fear, and manifold hegemonic forces (local and global) that jeopardize the possibility of experiencing genuine alternatives or making a full range of choices. This is the case for people whose kidneys sell on the global market, those who are caught in the transnational webs of human trafficking, or those whose environments, bodies, and imaginations have become polluted by progress and developmental agendas in which they are unable to participate or benefit. Many of us are also victims of perpetually whetted desires for consumer goods, new technologies, and the latest biomedical products, from a pair of perfect breasts and expensive intestinal worms to pharmaceutical neuroenhancers. We are at times victims of our global sweet tooth and our insatiable appetite for novelty and excess, our incessant quest for simple solutions to complex problems, as well as the modernist illusion that we may somehow soon conquer the indeterminacy of life and death by classifying and organizing every possible "thing" into neat nonoverlapping categories. We are also victims of the hope or expectation that hard evidence can fully unravel the mystery of how human bodies, minds, emotions, and the senses work together in life, dreams, illness, and even death.

It may be a legitimate and certainly a "rational" desire to wish to definitively settle which healing method really works and which one does not in order to protect "citizens" and "consumers" from dangerous or deceitful practices that masquerade as healing. Undoubtedly, there are some people cashing out on (s)CAMs, posing as healers to sell overpriced and low-quality services or goods, even toxic or contaminated "natural health products," to an ever-eager general public looking for wellness, healing, and hope. As consumers, philosophers, or co-creators of this polyphony of healing possibilities, we can be naïve, opportunistic, or passive in our engagement and response to the unending abundance of options in the global marketplace. Personal struggles and social injustices, along with moods and practical necessities frequently conspire to thwart our freedoms of self-care, participation, and social responsibility. Yet this is an opportune time to prevent, transform, and cure illness, to become more soulful, more mindful, and more embodied, to turn waste into food for the earth, and take responsibility for participation in the world. As we try to classify and sort out and integrate CAM into taxonomic classes and categories, old or new, we commit the fallacy of truncating them, as Cinderella's sisters chopped their toes and heels to make them fit into the perfect glass slippers. But what we have is the emergence and revision, production, and reproduction of a composite worldview and a new sensory and experiential spectrum of possibilities for healing that are by their nature contingent and intersubjective.

A provocative parable is the story of the Brazilian sorcerer Quesalid, told by Lévi-Strauss: a young man begins by mimicking the performance of healing, and to his surprise he becomes a sought-out healer whose patients are helped by his methods. Lévi-Strauss (1963:180) summarized the situation thusly: "Quesalid did not become a great shaman because he cured his patients; he cured his patients because he had become a great shaman." Reflecting on mimetic entanglements in the performance of healing, Jean Langford (1999) noted that Ayurvedic practitioners have sought legitimacy through imitation of European medicine, while folk practitioners have sought legitimacy through imitation of professional Ayurvedic doctors. Her informant, Dr. Mistry, represented himself as an Ayurvedic doctor, although his credentials and his elaborate method of pulse-reading were unconvincing. But during the course of her fieldwork with Dr. Mistry, Langford (1999:24, 40) understood that his pulse diagnosis was a first act of healing in his encounter with patients, "a sign of traditional wisdom," a gesture that "sparks the faith that fires the healing process." Amidst a quandary over quackery, she recognized this act as a divinatory process, which allowed the doctor to elicit the patients' complaints, not simply a source of factual information; the conversation which followed the pulse-taking allowing him to subsequently revise his assessment and engage the patient into the joint project of care and healing. Confessing that she frequently questioned Dr. Mistry's authenticity and needed to "discard one definition of quackery after another," Langford (1999:41) expanded on Michael Taussig's argument (1993) that *mimesis* accompanies every act of signification, including all forms of medicine, as health practitioners are trained through imitation and learn to use symbols and medicines to inspire trust. Ample evidence from all cultures points to the possibility of healing through simulation, which is the essence of the placebo effect, a prominent force in all traditions of medicine. Yet simulated healing is no less real and significant. Langford finds herself "recruited" in Dr. Mistry's self-promotion and validation enterprise when they are photographed together. I too found that my presence at certain events during my Romanian fieldwork was touted as evidence of the validity and global importance of the alternative medicine phenomenon, the ELTA movement in particular.

Practitioners of non-Western medical traditions seek legitimacy by imitating Western methods and formulae, and pursuing licensure and professionalization, while mainstream medical professionals seek to adopt, adapt, and absorb popular CAM practices that are evidence-based. Biomedical, complementary, or "alternative" practices and healing systems may not be neatly categorized and compartmentalized (segmented and segregated) by extraneous criteria rooted in preestablished Eurocentric frameworks of thought and health practice, as they are likely to perpetuate the limitations, constructions, and delimitations of mind, body, self, senses, materiality, and immateriality. Taxonomic exercises may be useful to carry out in practice, but inevitably a facile systematization entails significant distortions and misrepresentations of how "alternative" practices work and how they are experienced: fluidly and holistically, on social, emotional, physical, and metaphysical levels. Most practices blend all of the categories that are commonly (re)presented as distinct for governmental, administrative, or biomedical purposes.

Just as this book's chapter divisions do not represent impermeable categories of healing traditions, "alternative" healing approaches and practices criss-cross cognitive and experiential domains of contemporary life, blurring dominant notions and understandings of persons, relationships, and experiences. In the words of Jeremy Carrette and Richard King (2005:10): "Culture is a dynamic network of relations that can never be adequately represented by fixed categories." While familiar distinctions may be pragmatically useful, these scholars warn that "we should not be fooled[,] however[,] into believing that these abstractions somehow directly mirror the complexity of culture itself." Furthermore, cultural habits, embodied practices, and established thinking patterns may "prevent people from seeing both the interconnections of culture and power and also the ability of ideas to disrupt and challenge the established order" (Carrette and King 2005:11). I contend that it will be necessary to reconsider the cultural categories we publicly draw on to explore unorthodox and globalized healing methods in the coming decades. Substance-based therapies involve awareness and replenishment of vital forces, social and political networks, and energy resources; energy therapies involve embodied awareness, communication, and somatic modes of attention between practitioner and client; consciousness responds to sensations and movements of bodies and the biocultural flows, within and without persons and communities. These diverse forms of awareness, communication, interaction, and interrelation are not defined or bounded by prior analytical categories that our earnest planning efforts struggle to sort them into. This dynamic complexity exists because all healing alternatives emerged from unique historical and experiential intersections of cultures, environments, and biologies. Reality is much messier than our existing maps.

As complex societies embrace and evaluate novel schemas and possibilities of healing, traditional protocols of assessment will become confounded by unscripted states of awareness and the challenges of translating diverse alternative therapies into logical language and motion. We will inevitably encounter authenticity, mimetic hybridization, domestication, and quackery, too. It is a tremendously exciting time to be in the world: it tastes and smells like a millennial sort of time, when a new paradigm of healing is emerging in the West. We are required to re-soul and re-embody our senses and bodily boundaries, exploring new sensations and metaphors, emotions, and hidden spaces that originate in the re-foldings of self, ecology, and culture. Then we may experience an expanded universe of transformative paths to healing as they hatch their magical fruit.

References

Ackerman, Michael (2004), "Science and the Shadow of Ideology in the American Health Foods Movement, 1930s–1960s," in Robert D. Johnston (ed.), *The Politics of Healing: Histories of Alternative Medicine in Twentieth Century North America*, New York: Routledge.

Adams, Abigail E. (1998), "Gringas, Ghouls and Guatemala: The 1994 Attacks on North American Women Accused of Body Organ Trafficking," *Journal of Latin American Anthropology* 4(1): 112–33.

Adams, Glyn (2002), "Shiatsu in Britain and Japan: Personhood, Holism and Embodied Aesthetics," *Anthropology and Medicine* 9(3): 245–65.

Albanese, Catherine L. (1992), "The Magical Staff: Quantum Healing in the New Age," in J. R. Lewis and J. G. Melton (eds.), *Perspectives on the New Age*, Albany, NY: SUNY Press, pp. 68–84.

Alter, Joseph S. (1999), "Heaps of Health, Metaphysical Fitness: Ayurveda and the Ontology of Good Health in Medical Anthropology," *Current Anthropology* 40: 43–66.

aspencancerguide.org (2011), http://www.aspencancerguide.org/avh_aromatherapy.html, accessed April 10, 2011.

Baer, Hans A. (2001), *Biomedicine and Alternative Healing Systems in America: Issues of Class, Race, Ethnicity, and Gender*, Madison: University of Wisconsin Press.

Baer, Hans (2008), "The Emergence of Integrative Medicine in Australia: The Growing Interest of Biomedicine and Nursing in Complementary Medicine in a Southern Developed Society," *Medical Anthropology Quarterly* 22(1): 52–66.

Balzer, Marjorie Mandelstam (2006), "Sustainable Faith? Reconfiguring Shamanic Healing in Siberia," in J. Koss-Chioino and P. Hefner (eds.), *Spiritual Transformation and Healing: Anthropological, Technological, Neuroscientific and Clinical Perspectives*, Lanham, MD: AltaMira Press, pp. 78–100.

Boas, Franz (1911), *The Mind of Primitive Man*, New York: The Macmillan Company.

Boddy, Janice (1994), "Spirit Possession Revisited: Beyond Instrumentality," *Annual Reviews in Anthropology* 23: 407–34.

Bodeker, Gerard (2008), *Medicinal Plants for Forest Conservation and Health Care (FAO)*, New Delhi: Daya Publishing House.

Bodley, John (2007), *Anthropology and Contemporary Human Problems*, Lanham, MD: AltaMira Press.

Boeke, S. J., Boersma, M. G., Alink, G. M., van Loon, J. J., van Huis, A., Dicke, M., and Rietjens, I. M. (2004), "Safety Evaluation of Neem (*Azadirachta indica*), Derived Pesticides," *Journal of Ethnopharmacology* 94(1): 25–41.

Boia, Lucian (1998), "Cele două feţe ale mitologiei comuniste," in Lucian Boia (ed.), *Miturile comunismului românesc,* Bucureşti, România: Nemira, pp. 11–18.

Bourdieu, Pierre (1977), *Outline of a Theory of Practice,* Richard Nice (trans.), Stanford, CA: Stanford University Press.

Bourdieu, Pierre (1984), *Distinction: A Social Critique of the Judgment of Taste,* New York: Routledge.

Bourguignon, Erica (1968), *Cross-Cultural Study of Dissociational States,* Columbus: Ohio State University Press.

Bradley, James (2002), "Medicine on the Margins? Hydropathy and Orthodoxy in Britain, 1840–60," in Waltraud Ernst (ed.), *Plural Medicine, Tradition and Modernity, 1800–2000,* New York: Routledge, pp. 19–39.

Brahmachari G. (2004), "Neem—an Omnipotent Plant: A Retrospection," *Chembiochem: A European Journal of Chemical Biology* 5(4): 408–21.

Brown, Nell Porter (2010), "Easing Ills through Tai Chi: Researchers Study the Benefits of This Mind-Body Exercise," *Harvard Magazine* (Jan.–Feb.), http://harvardmagazine.com/2010/01/researchers-study-tai-chi-benefits, accessed April 11, 2011.

Buckle, Jane (2003), *Clinical Aromatherapy: Essential Oils in Practice,* 2nd ed., Philadelphia: Churchill Livingstone / Elsevier Science.

Bussmann, Rainer, and Sharon, Douglas (2006), "Traditional Medicinal Plant Use in Northern Peru: Tracking Two Thousand Years of Healing Culture," *Journal of Ethnobiology and Ethnomedicine* 2: 47.

Cant, Sarah, and Sharma, Ursula (1999), *A New Medical Pluralism? Alternative Medicine, Doctors, Patients and the State,* London: Routledge.

Carney, Scott (2010a), "Inside India's Rent-a-womb Business," *Mother Jones* (March–April), http://motherjones.com/politics/2010/02/surrogacy-tourism-india-nayna-patel.

Carney, Scott (2010b), "The Temple of Do," *Mother Jones* (March–April), http://motherjones.com/politics/2010/02/remy-hair-extensions-india.

Carrette, Jeremy, and King, Richard (2005), *Selling Spirituality: The Silent Takeover of Religion,* New York: Routledge.

Cassidy, Nigel (2011), "Herbal Remedies Face Licence Rules," BBC News Business (January 14), http://www.bbc.co.uk/news/business-12196371, accessed January 16, 2011.

Chen, Y., Kelton, C. M., Jing, Y., Guo, J. J., Li, X., and Patel, N. C. (2008), "Utilization, Price, and Spending Trends for Antidepressants in the US Medicaid Program," *Research in Social and Administrative Pharmacy* 4(3): 244–57.

Chirban, John T. (1991), "Healing and Spirituality," in J. Chirban (ed.), *Health and Faith: Medical, Psychological and Religious Dimensions*, Lanham, MD: University Press of America.

Classen, Constance (1992), "The Odor of the Other: Olfactory Symbolism and Cultural Categories," *Ethos* 20(2): 133–66.

ClinicalTrials.gov (2009), "Trichuris Suis Ova Adult Autism Symptom Domains (TSO)," http://clinicaltrials.gov/ct2/show/NCT01040221, accessed January 16, 2010.

Clottes, Jean, and Lewis-Williams, David (1998), *The Shamans of Prehistory: Trance and Magic in the Painted Caves,* New York: Harry N. Abrams.

Cohen, Elizabeth (2010), "Man Finds Extreme Healing Eating Parasitic Worms," CNN Health—Empowered Patient (Dec. 9), http://www.cnn.com/2010/HEALTH/12/09/worms.health/index.html, accessed January 16, 2011.

Comaroff, Jean (1985), *Body of Power, Spirit of Resistance: The Culture and History of a South African People,* Chicago: University of Chicago Press.

Comaroff, Jean, and Comaroff, John L. (1993), "Introduction," in J. Comaroff and J. Comaroff (eds.), *Modernity and Its Malcontents, Ritual and Power in Postcolonial Africa,* Chicago: University of Chicago Press, pp. xi–xxxvii.

Conrad, Peter (2007), *The Medicalization of Society: On the Transformation of Human Conditions into Treatable Disorders,* Baltimore, MD: The Johns Hopkins University Press.

Counihan, Carole, and Penny Van Esterik, eds. (1997), *Food and Culture: A Reader,* New York: Routledge.

Crandon-Malamud, Libbet (1991), *From the Fat of our Souls: Social Change, Political Process and Medical Pluralism in Bolivia,* Berkeley: University of California Press.

Csordas, Thomas J. (1990), "Embodiment as a Paradigm for Anthropology," *Ethos* 18: 5–47.

Csordas, Thomas J. (1997 [1994]), *The Sacred Self: A Cultural Phenomenology of Charismatic Healing,* Berkeley: University of California Press.

CU School of Medicine (2011), "Creighton Medical Students Introduced to Alternative Medicine," http://medschool.creighton.edu/medicine/departments/pharmacology/pharm/introtoalternativemed/, accessed January 12, 2011.

CUMC (2009a), "Online Resources—Complementary and Alternative Medicine," http://creightonhospital.staywellsolutionsonline.com/RelatedItems/85,P00188, accessed January 12, 2011.

CUMC (2009b), "Types of Complementary and Alternative Medicine," http://creightonhospital.staywellsolutionsonline.com/Library/News/85,P00189, accessed January 12, 2011.

Danforth, Loring M. (1989), *Firewalking and Religious Healing: The Anastenari of Greece and the American Firewalking Movement,* Princeton, NJ: Princeton University Press.

Davis-Floyd, Robbie E. (2004), *Birth as an American Rite of Passage,* Berkeley, CA: University of California Press.

Devisch, René (1993), *Weaving the Threads of Life: The Khita Gyn-Eco-Logical Healing Cult among the Yaka,* Chicago: University of Chicago Press.

Dobkin de Rios, Marlene (1984), *Hallucinogens: Cross-cultural Perspective,* Albuquerque: University of New Mexico Press.

Douglas, Mary (1966), *Purity and Danger: An Analysis of Concepts of Pollution and Taboo,* New York: Praeger.

Douglas, Mary (1970), *Natural Symbols: Explorations in Cosmology,* New York: Pantheon Books (Random House).

Douglas, Mary (1993), "The Forbidden Animals in Leviticus," *Journal for the Study of the Old Testament* 59: 3–23.

Douglas, Mary, and Isherwood, Baron (1996 [1979]), *The World of Goods: Towards an Anthropology of Consumption,* New York: Routledge.

Dream Online (2009), "Alternative Therapies," *Dream Online: A Magazine for Patients and Families,* Children's Hospital Boston, http://www.childrenshospital. org/dream/fall09/alternative_therapies_qa.html, accessed July 10, 2010.

Drewal, Henry John (2008), "Mami Wata: Arts for Water Spirits in Africa and Its Diaspora," *African Arts* 41(2): 60–83, http://www.mitpressjournals.org/doi/ abs/10.1162/afar.2008.41.2.60?journalCode=afar.

Durkheim, Émile (1965 [1915]), *The Elementary Forms of Religious Life,* New York: Free Press.

Ehrenreich, Barbara, and Hochschild, Arlie Russell (eds.) (2002), *Global Woman: Nannies, Maids, and Sex Workers in the New Economy,* New York: Henry Holt.

Eisenberg, David M., Kessler, Ronald C., Foster, Cindy, Norlock, Frances E., Calkins, David R., and Delblanco, Thomas L. (1993), "Unconventional Medicine in the United States: Prevalence, Costs, and Patterns of Use," *New England Journal of Medicine* 328(4): 246–52.

Eliade, Mircea (1991 [1954]), *The Myth of Eternal Return, Or, Cosmos and History,* Princeton, NJ: Princeton University Press.

Eliade, Mircea (2004 [1951]), *Shamanism: Archaic Techniques of Ecstasy,* Princeton, NJ: Princeton University Press.

Ellwood, Robert (1992), "How New is the New Age?" in J. R. Lewis and J. G. Melton (eds.), *Perspectives on the New Age,* Albany, NY: SUNY Press, pp. 59–67.

Ellwood, Wayne (2008), "This Toxic Life," *New Internationalist* 415(September), http://www.newint.org/features/2008/09/01/keynote-plastic/.

Eltauniversitate.ro (2011), Elta Universitate Romania, Official website, www. eltauniversitate.ro, accessed August 31, 2011.

Ernst, Waltraud (2002), *Plural Medicine, Tradition and Modernity, 1800–2000,* New York: Routledge.

Etkin, Nina L. (2006), *Edible Medicines: An Ethnopharmacology of Food,* Tucson: The University of Arizona Press.

Evans-Pritchard, Edward E. (1976 [1937]), *Witchcraft, Oracles and Magic among the Azande,* Oxford University Press.

Evseev, Ivan (1994), *Dicţionar de Simboluri si Arhetipuri Culturale,* Timişoara: Editura AMARCORD.

Fadiman, Anne (1997), *The Spirit Catches You and You Fall Down: A Hmong Child, Her American Doctors, and the Collision of Two Cultures,* New York: Farrar, Strauss and Giroux.

FAO (Food and Agriculture Organization of the United Nations) (2000), "The State of Food Insecurity in the World 2000," http://www.fao.org/DOCREP/X8200E/X8200E00.HTM, accessed July 23, 2010.

Farr, Kathryn (2004), *Sex Trafficking: The Global Market in Women and Children,* New York: Worth Publishers.

Farrer, Claire (2011 [1994]), *Thunder Rides a Black Horse: Mescalero Apaches and The Mythic Present,* Long Grove, IL: Waveland Press.

Foster, George M., and Anderson, Barbara Gallatin (1978), *Medical Anthropology,* New York: John Wiley & Sons.

Foucault, Michel (1988 [1965]), *Madness and Civilization: A History of Insanity in the Age of Reason,* New York: Random House.

Foucault, Michel (1988), "Technologies of the Self," in L. Martin, H. Gutman, and P. Hutton (eds.), *Technologies of the Self: A Seminar with Michel Foucault,* Amherst: University of Massachusetts Press, pp. 16–49.

Foucault, Michel (1994 [1973]), *The Birth of the Clinic: An Archaeology of Medical Perception,* New York: Random House.

Foucault, Michel (1997 [1984]), "The Ethics of the Concern of the Self as a Practice of Freedom," in P. Rabinow (ed.) and R. Hurley et al. (trans.), *Ethics: Subjectivity and Truth, by Michel Foucault,* New York: The New Press, pp. 281–301.

Frank, Arthur W. (2002), *At the Will of the Body: Reflections on Illness,* New York: Mariner Books.

Frank, Robert, and Ecks, Stefan (2004), "Towards an Ethnography of Indian Homeopathy," *Anthropology and Medicine* 11(3): 307–26.

Frazer, Sir James George (2000 [1922]), *The Golden Bough,* New York: Bartleby. com, http://www.bartleby.com/196/, accessed April 10, 2011.

Gadsby, Patricia (2004), "The Inuit Paradox," *Discover: Science, Technology, and The Future* (October 1), http://discovermagazine.com/2004/oct/inuit-paradox/article_print, accessed January 8, 2011.

Gauld, Alan (1992), *A History of Hypnotism,* Cambridge: Cambridge University Press.

Geertz, Clifford (1973), *The Interpretation of Cultures,* New York: HarperCollins.

Geurts, Kathryn Linn (2002), *Culture and the Senses: Bodily Ways of Knowing in an African Community,* Berkeley: University of California Press.

Gevitz, Norman (1988), *Other Healers: Unorthodox Medicine in America,* Baltimore: The Johns Hopkins University Press.

Ginsburg, Faye D., Abu-Lughod, Lila, and Larkin, Brian (2002), *Media Worlds: Anthropology on New Terrain,* Berkeley: University of California Press.

Gladney, Dru (1996), *Muslim Chinese: Ethnic Nationalism in the People's Republic,* 2nd ed., Cambridge, MA: Harvard University Asia Center.

Glass-Coffin, Bonnie (2010), "Shamanism and San Pedro through Time: Some Notes on the Archaeology, History and Continued Use of an Entheogen in Northern Peru," *Anthropology of Consciousness* 21(1): 58–82.

Gmelch, George (1978), "Baseball Magic," *Human Nature* 1(8): 32–40.

Good, Byron J. (1994), *Medicine, Rationality, and Experience: An Anthropological Perspective,* Cambridge, MA: Cambridge University Press.

Goodman, Felicitas D. (1988), *Ecstasy, Ritual, and Alternate Reaility: Religion in a Pluralistic World,* Bloomington: Indiana University Press.

Goodman, Felicitas D. (1990), *Where the Spirits Ride the Wind: Trance Journeys and Other Ecstatic Experiences,* Bloomington: Indiana University Press.

Gorski, Timothy N. (1999), "Do the Eisenberg Data Hold Up?" *The Scientific Review of Alternative Medicine* 3(2), http://www.sram.org/0302/eisenberg.html, accessed July 10, 2010.

Gouk, Penelope (ed.) (2000), *Musical Healing in Cultural Contexts,* Burlington, VT: Ashgate Publishers.

Green, Richard E. et al. (2010), "A Draft Sequence of the Neandertal Genome," *Science* 328(5979): 710–22, http://www.sciencemag.org/cgi/content/abstract/328/5979/710.

Greenfield, Sidney (2008), *Spirits with Scalpels: The Cultural Biology of Religious Healing in Brazil,* Walnut Creek, CA: Left Coast Press.

Greenwood, Susan (2009), *The Anthropology of Magic,* Oxford: Berg Publishers.

Hackett, Rosalind I. J. (1992), "New Age Trends in Nigeria: Ancestral or Alien Religion?" in J. R. Lewis and J. G. Melton (eds.), *Perspectives on the New Age,* Albany, NY: SUNY Press, pp. 215–231.

Hall, John R. (1979), "Apocalypse at Jonestown," *Society* 16: 52–61.

Halliburton, Murphy (2009), *Mudpacks and Prozac: Experiencing Ayurvedic, Biomedical, and Religious Healing,* Walnut Creek, CA: West Coast Press.

Harish Kumar, G., Vidya Priyadarsini, R., Vinothini, G., Vidjaya Letchoumy, P., and Nagini, S. (2010), "The Neem Limonoids Azadirachtin and Nimbolide Inhibit Cell Proliferation and Induce Apoptosis in an Animal Model of Oral Oncogenesis," *Investigational New Drugs* 28(4): 392–401.

Harper, Janice (2002), *Endangered Species: Health, Illness, and Death among Madagascar's People of the Forest,* Durham, NC: Carolina Academic Press.

Harris, Marvin (1989 [1974]), *Cows, Pigs, Wars and Witches: The Riddles of Culture,* New York: Vintage.

Hinojosa, Servando (2002), "'The Hands Know': Bodily Engagement and Medical Impasse in Highland Maya Bonesetting," *Medical Anthropology Quarterly* 16(1): 22–40.

Hinton, Devon E., Howes, David, and Kirmayer, Laurence J. (2008), "Toward a Medical Anthropology of Sensations: Definitions and Research Agenda," *Transcultural Psychiatry* 45(2): 142–62.

Hobday, Richard (1999), *The Healing Sun: Sunlight and Health in the 21st Century,* Forres, UK: Findhorn Press.

Holt-Lunstad, J., Smith, T. B., and Layton, J. B. (2010), "Social Relationships and Mortality Risk: A Meta-Analytic Review," *PLoS Med.* 77(7): e1000316, http://www.ncbi.nlm.nih.gov/pubmed/20668659, accessed January 22, 2011.

Horwitz, Allan V. (2002), *Creating Mental Illness,* Chicago: University of Chicago Press.

Hover-Kramer, Dorothea (2002), *Healing Touch: A Guidebook for Practitioners,* 2nd ed., Albany, NY: Delmar/Thomson Learning.

Howes, David (2005), "Hyperaesthesia, or, the Sensual Logic of Late Capitalism," in D. Howes (ed.), *The Empire of the Senses: The Sensual Culture Reader,* Oxford: Berg.

Hpathy.com (2011), http://hpathy.com/homeopathic-interviews/, accessed April 15, 2011.

Hsu, Elizabeth (1999), *The Transmission of Chinese Medicine,* Cambridge: Cambridge University Press.

Hsu, Elizabeth (2002), "'The Medicine from China Has Rapid Effects': Chinese Medicine Patients in Tanzania," *Anthropology and Medicine* 9(3): 291–313.

Illich, Ivan (1976), *Medical Nemesis: The Expropriation of Health,* New York: Pantheon Books.

Janzen, John M. (2002), *The Social Fabric of Health: An Introduction to Medical Anthropology,* New York: McGraw-Hill.

Johnston, Barbara Rose (ed.) (1994), *Who Pays the Price? The Sociocultural Context of Environmental Crisis,* Washington, DC: Island Press.

Johnston, R. D. (ed.) (2004), *The Politics of Healing: Histories of Alternative Medicine in Twentieth-Century North America,* New York: Routledge.

Jordan, Brigitte, with Davis-Floyd, Robbie (1992), *Birth in Four Cultures: A Crosscultural Investigation of Childbirth in Yucatan, Holland, Sweden, and the United States,* Prospect Heights, IL: Waveland Press.

Joseph, R. (1988), "The Right Cerebral Hemisphere: Emotion, Music, Visual-Spatial Skills, Body-Image, Dreams, and Awareness," *Journal of Clinical Psychology* 44(5): 630–73.

Katz, Richard (1982), *Boiling Energy: Community Healing Among the Kalahari Kung,* Boston: Harvard University Press.

Kaufman, Suzanne D. (2005), *Consuming Visions: Mass Culture and the Lourdes Shrine,* Ithaca, NY: Cornell University Press.

Keegan, Lynn (2001), *Healing with Complementary and Alternative Therapies,* Albany, NY: Delmar (Thomson Learning).

Kerr, Catherine (2002), "Translating 'Mind-in-Body': Two Models of Patient Experience Underlying a Randomized Controlled Trial of Qigong," *Culture, Medicine and Psychiatry* 26: 419–47.

Kersiek, Kristen (2008), "Parasites—The Uninvited Dinner Guests," *Infection Research* (Oct. 15), http://www.infection-research.de/perspectives/detail/pressrelease/parasites_the_uninvited_dinner_guests-1/, accessed April 10, 2011.

Khalsa, Soram (2009), *The Vitamin D Revolution: How the Power of This Amazing Vitamin Can Change Your Life,* New York: Hay House.

Kirmayer, Laurence J. (1992), "The Body's Insistence on Meaning: Metaphor as Presentation and Representation in Illness Experience," *Medical Anthropology Quarterly* 6(4): 323–46.

Klass, Morton (1995), *Ordered Universes: Approaches to the Anthropology of Religion,* Boulder, CO: Westview Press.

Klassen, Pamela E. (2001), *Blessed Events: Religion and Home Birth in America,* Princeton, NJ: Princeton University Press.

Kleinman, Arthur (1986), *Social Origins of Distress and Disease: Depression, Neurasthenia and Pain in Modern China,* New Haven, CT: Yale University Press.

Kleinman, Arthur (1988), *The Illness Narratives: Suffering, Healing, and the Human Condition,* New York: Basic Books.

Kleinman, Arthur (1995), *Writing at the Margin: Discourse between Anthropology and Medicine,* Berkeley: University of California Press.

Kligman, Gail (1998), *The Politics of Duplicity: Controlling Reproduction in Ceausescu's Romania,* Berkeley: University of California Press.

Koen, Benjamin D. (2009), *Beyond the Roof of the World: Music, Prayer, and Healing in the Pamir Mountains,* New York: Oxford University Press.

Koen, Benjamin D., with Lloyd, Jacqueline, Barz, Gregory, and Brummel-Smith, Karen (2009), *The Oxford Handbook of Medical Ethnomusicology,* New York: Oxford University Press.

Korsmeyer, Carolyn (2002), *Making Sense of Taste,* Ithaca, NY: Cornell University Press.

Krieger, Dolores (1979), *The Therapeutic Touch: How to Use Your Hands to Help or to Heal,* Englewood Cliffs, NJ: Prentice-Hall.

Kuhn, Thomas (1996 [1962]), *The Structure of Scientific Revolutions,* Chicago: The University of Chicago Press.

Kuriyama, Shigehisa (2002), *The Expressiveness of the Body and the Divergence of Greek and Chinese Medicine,* New York: Zone Books.

Lakoff, Andrew (2005), *Pharmaceutical Reason: Knowledge and Value in Global Psychiatry,* Cambridge Studies in Society and Life Sciences, Cambridge: Cambridge University Press.

Langford, Jean M. (1999), "Medical Mimesis: Healing Signs of a Cosmopolitan 'Quack,'" *American Ethnologist* 26(1): 24–46.

Lázár, Imre (2006), "Táltos Healers, Neoshamans and Multiple Medical Realities in Hungary," in H. Johannessen and I. Lázár (eds.), *Multiple Medical Realities: Patients and Healers in Biomedical, Alternative and Traditional Medicine*, New York: Berghahn Books.

Lee, Richard B. (2003), *The Dobe Ju/'hoansi,* 3rd ed., Belmont, CA: Wadsworth/ Cengage Learning.

Lee-Treweek, Geraldine, Heller, Tom, Spurr, Susan, MacQueen, Hilary, and Katz, Jeanne (eds.) (2005), *Perspectives on Complementary and Alternative Medicine: A Reader*, New York: Routledge.

Leguit, P. (2004), "Hospital as a Temple," *Patient Education and Counseling* 53(1): 27–30.

Lévi-Strauss, Claude (1963), *Structural Anthropology,* New York: Basic Books.

Lie, John (2004), *Multiethnic Japan,* Boston: Harvard University Press.

Lim, Louisa (2009), "Swine Flu Bumps Up Price of Chinese Spice," NPR (May 18), http://www.npr.org/templates/story/story.php?storyId=104191227.

Lindquist, Galina (2006), *Conjuring Hope: Healing and Magic in Contemporary Russia,* New York: Berghahn Books.

Lock, Margaret (1980), *East Asian Medicine in Urban Japan: Varieties of Medical Experience,* Berkeley: University of California Press.

Lock, Margaret (1995), *Encounters with Aging: Mythologies of Menopause in Japan and North America*, Berkeley: University of California Press.

Lock, Margaret, and Scheper-Hughes, Nancy (1987), "The Mindful Body: A Prolegomenon to Future Work in Medical Anthropology," *Medical Anthropology Quarterly* 1(1): 6–41.

London, William M. (2006), "Newsweek's Misleading Report on 'Alternative Medicine,'" Quackwatch.org, http://www.quackwatch.org/04ConsumerEducation/ newsweek.html, accessed July 10, 2010.

Lorenz, Hendrik (2009), "Ancient Theories of Soul," in Edward N. Zalta (ed.), *The Stanford Encyclopedia of Philosophy (Summer 2009 Edition)*, http://plato. stanford.edu/archives/sum2009/entries/ancient-soul/.

Malinowski, Bronislaw (1920), "Kula: The Circulating Exchange of Valuables in the Archipelagoes of Eastern New Guinea," *Man* 20(51): 97–105.

Malinowski, Bronislaw (1935), *Coral Gardens and Their Magic*, New York: Dover.

Malinowski, Bronislaw (1992 [1948]), *Magic, Science and Religion and Other Essays,* Prospect Heights, IL: Waveland Press.

Marcus, George, and Fischer, Michael (1986), *Anthropology as Cultural Critique.* Chicago: University of Chicago Press.

Marshall Thomas, Elizabeth (1989 [1958]), *The Harmless People,* New York: Vintage Books.

Martin, Emily (1994), *Flexible Bodies: The Role of Immunity in American Culture from the Days of Polio to the Age of AIDS,* Boston: Beacon Press

Martin, Emily (2001), *The Woman in the Body: A Cultural Analysis of Reproduction,* rev. ed., Boston: Beacon Press.

Martin, Emily (2009), *Bipolar Expeditions: Mania and Depression in American Culture,* Princeton, NJ: Princeton University Press.

Masquelier, Adeline (2001), *Prayer Has Spoiled Everything: Possession, Power, and Identity in an Islamic Town of Niger,* Durham, NC: Duke University Press.

Mauss, Marcel (1972), *A General Theory of Magic,* R. Brain (trans.), New York: W. W. Norton [Original work published in 1902–1903].

Mauss, Marcel (1973), "Techniques of the Body," *Economy and Society* 2(1): 70–78.

Mauss, Marcel (1990 [1950, 1925]), *The Gift,* New York: W. W. Norton.

McClellan, Randall (1991), *The Healing Forces of Music: History, Theory and Practice,* Rockport, MA: Element Books.

Merleau-Ponty, Maurice (1962), *Phenomenology of Perception,* Colin Smith (trans.), London: Routledge and Kegan Paul.

Merriam-Webster's Online Dictionary (2010), http://mw4.m-w.com/dictionary/.

Miller, Daniel (1998), *A Theory of Shopping,* Ithaca, NY: Cornell University Press.

Mintz, Sidney (1985), *Sweetness and Power: The Place of Sugar in Modern History,* New York: Penguin.

Moerman, Daniel (2000), "Cultural Variations in the Placebo Effect: Ulcers, Anxiety, and Blood Pressure," *Medical Anthropology Quarterly* 14(1): 51–72.

Moerman, Daniel (2002), *Meaning, Medicine and the "Placebo Effect,"* Cambridge: Cambridge University Press.

NCCAM (2011), The National Center for Complementary and Alternative Medicine, http://nccam.nih.gov/.

NCCAM Tai Chi (2011), *Tai Chi,* http://nccam.nih.gov/health/taichi/, accessed April 10, 2011.

Needham, Rodney (1975), "Polythetic Classification: Convergence and Consequences," *Man* 10: 349–69.

Novella, Steven (2007), "The Golden Age of Quackery and Anti-Science," *The Scientific Review of Alternative Medicine* 11, http://www.sram.org/1101/goldenage.html, accessed July 10, 2010.

Ohnuki-Tierney, Emiko (1984), *Illness and Culture in Contemporary Japan: An Anthropogical View,* Cambridge: Cambridge University Press.

Olafson, Frederick A. (2010), "Philosophical Anthropology," *Encyclopædia Britannica Online,* http://www.britannica.com/EBchecked/topic/456743/philosophical-anthropology, accessed December 31, 2010.

O'Neil, Dennis (2006), "Explanations of Illness," http://anthro.palomar.edu/medical/med_1.htm, accessed October 30, 2010.

Oosthuizen, Gehardus C. (1992), "The 'Newness' of the New Age in South Africa and Reactions to It," in J. R. Lewis and J. G. Melton (eds.), *Perspectives on the New Age,* Albany, NY: SUNY Press, pp. 247–270.

Osher (2011), "Neuroscience of Meditation, Healing and the Sense of Touch," http://www.osher.hms.harvard.edu/kerrlab/what_we_study.html.

Owen, David (2007), *Principles and Practice of Homeopathy: The Therapeutic and Healing Process,* Philadelphia: Churchill Livingstone/Elsevier Health Sciences.

Pandian, Jacob (1991), *Culture, Religion, and the Sacred Self: A Critical Introduction to the Anthropological Study of Religion,* Englewood Cliffs, NJ: Prentice Hall.

Parreñas, Rhacel Salazar (2001), *Servants of Globalization: Women, Migration and Domestic Work,* Stanford, CA: Stanford University Press.

Paxson, Heather (2008), "Post-Pasteurian Cultures: The Microbiopolitics of Raw-Milk Cheese in the United States," *Cultural Anthropology* 23(1): 15–47.

Pollack, Andrew (2009), "Is Money Tainting the Plasma Supply?" *The New York Times* (December 5), http://www.nytimes.com/2009/12/06/business/06plasma.html, accessed August 8, 2010.

Pollan, Michael (2006), *The Omnivore's Dilemma: A Natural History of Four Meals,* New York: Penguin Books.

Porter, P. W. (2001), "Cultural Ecology," in N. J. Smelser and P. B. Baltes (eds.), *International Encyclopedia of the Social and Behavioral Sciences,* Oxford: Elsevier.

Price, Shirley, and Price, Len (1999), *Aromatherapy for Health Professionals,* 2nd ed., London: Churchill Livingstone.

Priyadarsini, R. V., Murugan, R. S., Sripriya, P., Karunagaran, D., and Nagini, S. (2010), "The Neem Limonoids Azadirachtin and Nimbolide Induce Cell Cycle Arrest and Mitochondria-Mediated Apoptosis in Human Cervical Cancer (HeLa), Cells," *Free Radical Research* 44(6): 624–34.

Quanten, Patrick (2002), "Healing vs. Curing," http://freespace.virgin.net/ahcare.qua/literature/mindspirit/healingvscuring.html, accessed January 4, 2010.

Rapp, Rayna (2000), *Testing Women, Testing the Fetus: The Social Impact of Amniocentesis in America (The Anthropology of Everydaylife),* New York: Routledge.

Rappaport, Roy A. (1968), *Pigs for the Ancestors: Ritual in the Ecology of a New Guinea People,* New Haven, CT: Yale University Press.

Ray, Celeste (2010), "Ireland's Holy Wells: Healing Waters and Contested Liturgies," *Anthropology News* 51(2): 8–11 (February 2010).

Reichel-Dolmatoff, G. (1976), "Cosmology as Ecological Analysis: A View from the Rain Forest," *Man* 11(3): 307–18.

Romanucci-Ross, Lola (1969), "The Hierarchy of Resort in Curative Practices: The Admiralty Island," *Journal of Health and Social Behavior* 10: 201–9.

Rosaldo, Renato (1989), *Culture and Truth: The Remaking of Social Analysis,* Boston: Beacon Press.

Roseman, Marina (1993), *Healing Sounds from the Malaysian Rainforest: Temiar Music and Medicine,* Berkeley: University of California Press.

Ross, Anamaria (2003), *Healing, Orthodoxy and Personhood in Postsocialist Romania,* PhD dissertation, Tulane University, UMI Company, www.il.proquest.com.

Rossi, Ernest L. (2002), *The Psychobiology of Gene Expression: Neuroscience and Neurogenesis in Hypnosis and the Healing Arts,* New York: W. W. Norton.

Roth, Mark (2006), "Some Women May See 100 Million Colors, Thanks to Their Genes," *Pittsburg Post-Gazette* (Sep. 13), http://www.post-gazette.com/pg/06256/721190–114.stm, accessed April 11, 2011.

Rowley, Michelle (2010), "Worms to My Rescue! The Story of Me and My 70 New Best Friends: Hookworms y'all," http://worms.michellerowley.com/, accessed January 16, 2011.

Săhleanu, Victor (1972), *Ştiinţa ţi Filozofia Informaţiei,* Bucureşti, Romania: Biblioteca de Filozofie şi Sociologie.

Salimpoor, Valorie N., Benovoy, Mitchel, Larcher, Kevin, Dagher, Alain, and Zatorre, Robert (2011), "Anatomically Distinct Dopamine Release during Anticipation and Experience of Peak Emotion to Music," *Nature Neuroscience* 14: 257–62.

Scheid, Volker (2002), *Chinese Medicine in Contemporary China: Plurality and Synthesis,* Durham, NC: Duke University Press.

Scheper-Hughes, Nancy (1996), "Theft of Life: The Globalization of Organ Stealing Rumours," *Anthropology Today* 12(3): 3–11.

Scheper-Hughes, Nancy, and Lock, Margaret (1987), "The Mindful Body: A Prolegomenon to Future Work in Medical Anthropology," *Medical Anthropology Quarterly* 1: 6–41.

Scheper-Hughes, Nancy, and Wacquant, Loïc (2002), *Commodifying Bodies,* London: Sage Publications.

Schmahl, G., Al-Rasheid, K. A., Abdel-Ghaffar, F., Klimpel, S., and Mehlhorn, H. (2010), "The Efficacy of Neem Seed Extracts (Tre-san, MiteStop on a Broad Spectrum of Pests and Parasites," *Parasitology Research* 107(2): 261–69.

Schultes, Richard Evans, Hofmann, Albert, and Rätsch, Christian (2001), *Plants of the Gods: Their Sacred, Healing, and Hallucinogenic Powers,* Rochester, VT: Healing Arts Press.

Scott, Robert (2010), *Miracle Cures: Saints, Pilgrimage and the Healing Power of Belief,* Berkeley: University of California Press.

SF (2011), Slow Food International, www.slowfood.com, accessed April 2, 2011.

Sharp, Lesley (1996), *The Possessed and the Dispossessed: Spirits, Identity, and Power in a Madagascar Migrant Town,* Berkeley: University of California Press.

Shiva, Vandana (2000), *Stolen Harvest: The Hijacking of the Global Food Supply,* Cambridge, MA: South End Press.

Siegel, Bernie S. (1990 [1986]), *Love, Medicine and Miracles: Lessons Learned about Self-Healing from a Surgeon's Experience with Exceptional Patients,* New York: Harper Perennial.

Singer, Merrill, and Baer, Hans (2007), *Introducing Medical Anthropology: A Discipline in Action*, Lanham, MD: AltaMira Press.

Snyder, Solomon H. (2008), "Seeking God in the Brain—Efforts to Localize Higher Brain Functions," *New England Journal of Medicine* 358: 6–7.

Sontag, Susan (1990), *Illness as Metaphor and AIDS and Its Metaphors,* New York: Doubleday.

Spector, Ferrinne, and Maurer, Daphne (2009), "Synesthesia: A New Approach to Understanding the Development of Perception," *Developmental Psychology* 45(1): 175–89.

Stoller, Paul (1997), *Sensuous Scholarship,* Philadelphia: University of Pennsylvania Press.

Strachan, David P. (1989), "Hay Fever, Hygiene, and Household Size," *British Medical Journal* 299(6710): 1259–60.

Strassman, Rick (2000), *DMT: The Spirit Molecule: A Doctor's Revolutionary Research into the Biology of Near-Death and Mystical Experiences,* Rochester, VT: Park St. Press.

Stratan, Lucian (1997), *Boala: Invenția Civilizației Umane, Manualul Îngerului, Volumul VI,* București: Asociația Elta Universitate.

Strathern, Andrew J. (1996), *Body Thoughts.* Ann Arbor: University of Michigan Press.

Strathern, Andrew, and Stewart, Pamela (1999), *Curing and Healing: Medical Anthropology in Global Perspective,* Durham, NC: Carolina Academic Press.

Subapriya, R., and Nagini, S. (2005), "Medicinal Properties of Neem Leaves: A Review," *Current Medicinal Chemistry, Anticancer Agents* 5(2): 149–56.

Sutton, David E. (2001), *Remembrance of Repasts: An Anthropology of Food and Memory,* New York: Berg.

Tambiah, Stanley (1968), "The Magical Power of Words," *Man* 3(2): 175–208.

Tambiah, Stanley (1979), "A Performative Approach to Ritual," Radcliffe-Brown Lecture, *Proceedings of the British Academy* 66: 113–69.

Taussig, Michael (1993), *Mimesis and Alterity: A Particular History of the Senses,* New York: Routledge.

Tedlock, Barbara. (2005), *The Woman in the Shaman's Body: Reclaiming the Feminine in Religion and Medicine,* New York: Bantam.

Tett, Gillian (2009), "Icebergs and Ideologies: How Information Flows Fuelled the Financial Crisis," *Anthropology News* 50: 6–7.

Thakurta, P., Bhowmik, P., Mukherjee, S., Hajra, T. K., Patra, A., and Bag, P. K. (2007), "Antibacterial, Antisecretory and Antihemorrhagic Activity of Azadirachta Indica Used to Treat Cholera and Diarrhea in India," *Journal of Ethnopharmacology* 111(3): 607–12.

Thompson, C. J. (1929), *The Mystery and Art of the Apothecary,* London: John Lane the Bodley Head.

TRI (2011), Touch Research Institute at the University of Miami Medical School, http://www6.miami.edu/touch-research/InfantMassage.html, accessed January 28, 2011.

Trimble, Michael (2007), *The Soul in the Brain: The Cerebral Basis of Language, Art, and Belief,* Baltimore: Johns Hopkins University Press.

Turner, Edith (2006), "The Making of a Shaman: A Comparative Study of Inuit, African, and Nepalese Shaman Initiation," in J. Koss-Chioino and P. Hefner (eds.), *Spiritual Transformation and Healing: Anthropological, Technological, Neuroscientific and Clinical Perspectives*, Lanham, MD: AltaMira Press.

Turner, Victor (1967), *The Forest of Symbols: Aspects of Ndembu Ritual,* Ithaca, NY: Cornell University Press.

Turner, Victor (1969), *The Ritual Process: Structure and Anti-Structure,* Chicago: Aldine Publishing.

Turner, Victor, and Turner, Edith (1978), *Image and Pilgrimage in Christian Culture,* New York: Columbia University Press.

Tylor, Edward Burnett (2009 [1903]), *Primitive Culture,* vol. 1, Ithaca, NY: Cornell University Library.

Ullman, Dana (1991 [1988]), *Discovering Homeopathy, Medicine for the 21st Century: Your Introduction to the Science and Art of Homeopathic Medicine,* Berkeley, CA: North Atlantic Books.

Urbanhomestead.org (2010), http://urbanhomestead.org/, accessed September 2010.

Van Hollen, Cecilia (2003), *Birth on the Threshold: Childbirth and Modernity in South India,* Berkeley: University of California Press.

Veatch, Robert (1972), "Medical Ethics: Professional or Universal," *Harvard Theological Review* 65: 531–59.

Verdery, Katherine (1991), *National Ideology under Socialism: Identity and Cultural Politics in Ceaușescu's Romania,* Berkeley: University of California Press.

Vogt, Evon Z., and Hyman, Ray (2000 [1959]), *Water Witching U.S.A.,* 2nd ed., Chicago: The University of Chicago Press.

Ware, Timothy (1993), *The Orthodox Church,* London: Penguin Books.

Ware, Timothy (1996), "'In the Image and Likeness': The Uniqueness of the Human Person," in J. Chirban (ed.), *Personhood: Orthodox Christianity and the Connection Between Body, Mind, and Soul,* Westport, CT: Bergin and Garvey, pp. 1–13.

Watson, Dave (2005), "What Is the Definition of Energy?" FT Exploring Science and Technology website, http://www.ftexploring.com/energy/definition.html, accessed July 16, 2010.

Weinstock, J. V., and Elliott, D. E. (2009), "Helminths and the IBD Hygiene Hypothesis," *Inflammatory Bowel Disease* 15(1): 128–33.

Weitz, Rose (2009), *The Sociology of Health, Illness and Health Care: A Critical Approach,* 5th ed., Boston: Wadsworth/Cengage Learning.

Whiteford, Michael B. (1999), "Homeopathic Medicine in the City of Oaxaca, Mexico: Patients' Perspectives and Observations," *Medical Anthropology Quarterly* 13(1): 69–78.

WHO (World Health Organization) (2001a), "Turning the Tide of Malnutrition: Responding to the Challenge of the 21st Century," NHD/WHO/00.7, www.who.int/mip2001/files/2232/NHDbrochure.pdf, accessed July 23, 2010.

WHO (World Health Organization) (2001b), "Water-Related Diseases," http://www.who.int/water_sanitation_health/diseases/malnutrition/en/, accessed July 23, 2010.

WHO (World Health Organization) (2010), "Nutrition for Health and Development," http://www.who.int/nutrition/en/, accessed July 23, 2010.

Whorton, James C. (2002), *Nature Cures: The History of Alternative Medicine in America,* New York: Oxford University Press.

Williams, Michele A. (2004), *Only the Essentials,* Los Alamos, CA: Aroma Rx.

Winkelman, Michael (1991), "Therapeutic Effects of Hallucinogens," *The Anthropology of Consciousness* 2(3–4): 15–19.

Winkelman, Michael (1994), "Multidisciplinary Perspectives on Consciousness," *Anthropology of Consciousness* 5: 16–25.

Winkelman, Michael (2000), *Shamanism: The Neural Ecology of Consciousness and Healing,* Westport, CT: Bergin and Garvey.

Winkelman, Michael (2001a), "Psychointegrators: Multidisciplinary Perspectives on the Therapeutic Effects of Hallucinogens," *Complementary Health Practice Review* 6(3): 219–37.

Winkelman, Michael (2001b), "Alternative and Traditional Medicine Approaches for Substance Abuse Programs: A Shamanic Perspective," *The International Journal of Drug Policy* 12(4): 337–51.

Yapko, Michael D. (2001), *Treating Depression with Hypnosis: Integrating Cognitive-Behavioral and Strategic Approaches,* Philadelphia: Brunner-Routledge.

Young, Allan (1982), "The Anthropologies of Illness and Sickness," *Annual Review of Anthropology* 11: 257–85.

Index

- aetiology
- Cultural context of illness/disease
- etiology

Made in the USA
Las Vegas, NV
10 August 2021